50 BEST SHORT HIKES
YOSEMITE
National Park
and Vicinity

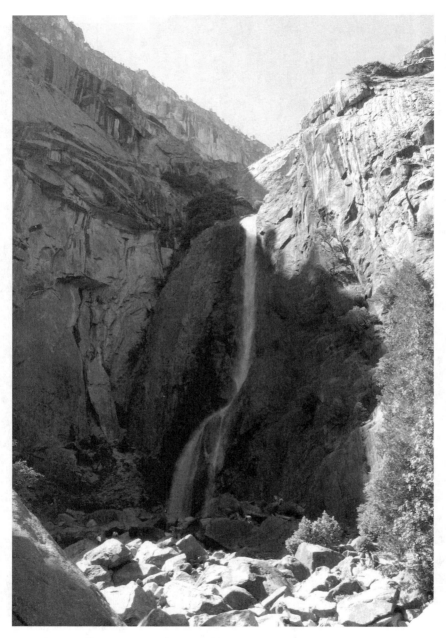

Lower Yosemite Fall in midsummer (see page 46)

50 BEST SHORT HIKES

YOSEMITE

National Park
and Vicinity

Elizabeth Wenk

 WILDERNESS PRESS . . . *on the trail since 1967*

50 Best Short Hikes Yosemite National Park and Vicinity

2nd EDITION 2012

Copyright © 2012 by Elizabeth Wenk

Front cover photo of Tioga Lake and back cover photo of middle Gaylor Lake
    copyright © by Elizabeth Wenk
Interior photos, except where noted, by Elizabeth Wenk
Maps and cover design: Scott McGrew
Interior design and layout: Annie Long
Editor: Amber Kaye Henderson

Library of Congress Cataloging-in-Publication Data

Wenk, Elizabeth.
  50 best short hikes Yosemite National Park and vicinity / Elizabeth Wenk. — 1st ed.
  p. cm.
  ISBN-13: 978-0-89997-631-0 (pbk.)
  ISBN-10: 0-89997-631-X ()
  1. Hiking—California—Yosemite National Park—Guidebooks. 2. Yosemite National Park
  (Calif.)—Guidebooks. I. Title. II. Title: Fifty best short hikes Yosemite National Park and
  vicinity.
  GV199.42.C22Y67987 2012
  917.94'47—dc23
                            2011053066

Manufactured in the United States of America

Published by: **Wilderness Press**
        c/o Keen Communications
        PO Box 43673
        Birmingham, AL 35243
        (800) 443-7227; FAX (205) 326-1012
        info@wildernesspress.com
        www.wildernesspress.com

Visit our website for a complete listing of our books and for ordering information.

Distributed by Publishers Group West

Safety Notice
Although Keen Communications/Wilderness Press and the author have made every attempt to ensure that the information in this book is accurate at press time, they are not responsible for any loss, damage, injury, or inconvenience that may occur to anyone while using this book. You are responsible for your own safety and health while in the wilderness. The fact that a trail is described in this book does not mean that it will be safe for you. Be aware that trail conditions can change from day to day. Always check local conditions, know your own limitations, and consult a map and compass.

Contents

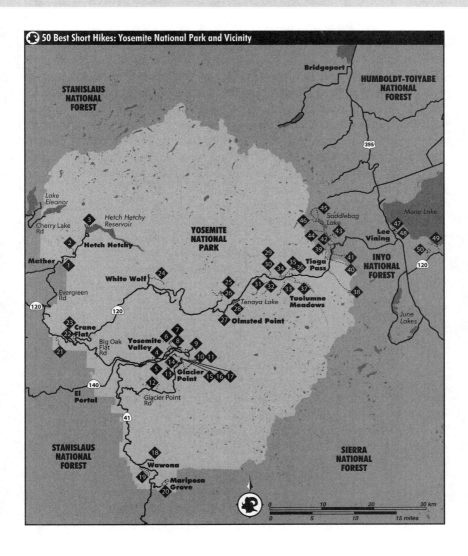

50 Best Short Hikes: Yosemite National Park and Vicinity

Acknowledgments

The offer to write this book arrived from Wilderness Press at a perfect time: I had 6-month-old and 2½-year-old daughters and was increasingly having fun exploring and reexploring the shorter trails in the Sierra. My husband, Douglas, and daughters, Eleanor and Sophia, supported me throughout the research for the hikes, obligingly following me down the trails or patiently waiting for me by a river play spot or pullout. Eleanor, just 5 now, has walked more than half the trails described here, and Sophia has accompanied me on nearly all of them, albeit in a backpack. Thanks as well to my sisters, Rebecca and Evelyn Wenk, and friends Louise Berben, Alisa Ellsworth, Cadie Hall, Charlotte Helvie, Candace and Eric Renger, Steven Thaw, John Williams, and others who also accompanied me on Yosemite walks over the last few years.

I acknowledge the many park service interpretive rangers and park scientists with whom I have spoken while writing this book. Each conversation has expanded my knowledge about Yosemite and the preservation of its natural resources. I also acknowledge the many people who have written books about Yosemite natural history and human history, for the more I learn, the more I appreciate Yosemite and see its secrets as I walk down the trail. The most important author to acknowledge is the grandfather of Yosemite, John Muir; I reread several of his books as I began writing, for in them is buried an incredible richness of natural history and a conservation ethic that was far ahead of its time.

The staff at Wilderness Press have been helpful and supportive throughout. As always I appreciate their flexibility in how I write the manuscript.

The Very Best Short Hikes

VERY BEST FOR LOCATION

VERY BEST FOR DESTINATION

VERY BEST FOR HISTORICAL INTEREST

VERY BEST FOR ALPINE SCENERY

39. Gaylor Lakes and Great Sierra Mine *Big alpine lakes, bright-green meadows, and striking views to the Cathedral Range*

41. Dana Plateau *Expansive views, steep escarpment, and alpine wildflowers*

43. Gardisky Lake *Alpine lake perched on a pass and flanked by accessible ridges; colorful meadows*

44. Slate Creek Fork of Lee Vining Creek *A magnificent backdrop featuring a semicircle of steep granite walls with year-round snowbanks*

45. Twenty Lakes Basin *Endless lakes and tarns, verdant meadows, and towering granite and metamorphic peaks*

VERY BEST FOR CHILDREN

8. Swinging Bridge and Superintendent's Bridge *Waterfall views, bridges, and boardwalks keep children engaged along this flat loop*

14. Sentinel Dome *One of Yosemite's easiest summit hikes*

29. Pothole Dome *Young children happily run up the slabs to the top*

30. Tuolumne River *Short walk to wonderful swimming holes and beaches*

VERY BEST LESS-TRAVELED

4. Base of El Capitan *Quiet location to absorb an immense granite wall*

21. Merced Grove *Peaceful forest walk to some wonderful sequoias you can enjoy in solitude*

44. Slate Creek Fork of Lee Vining Creek *Chance to wander past boulders and slab-dotted meadows and beneath tall ridges*

48. Lee Vining Creek *Location to quietly explore the Mono Basin, with Mono Lake views, aspen groves, and Lee Vining Creek*

VERY BEST FOR WILDFLOWERS

VERY BEST FOR WALKING ON GRANITE SLABS

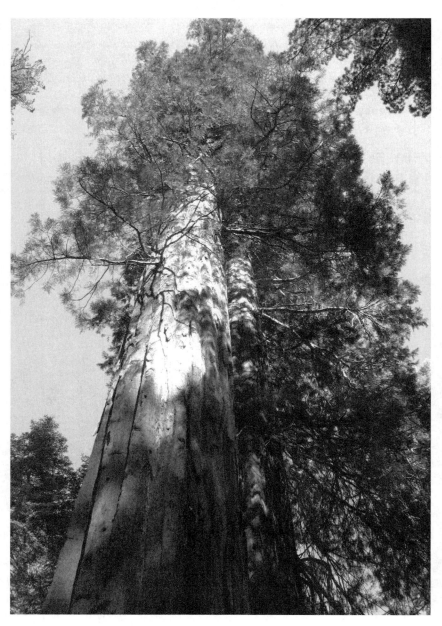

Giant sequoia in the Merced Grove (see page 109)

INTRODUCTION

Yosemite National Park is one of the country's best-known and most-visited national parks, with approximately 4 million visitors annually. Yosemite Valley is its most famous feature, with eight waterfalls, the sheer faces of Half Dome and El Capitan, and a grand collection of pinnacles, towers, and cliffs. However, Yosemite Valley occupies just a fraction of the national park, and Yosemite's treasures are much more diverse. A visitor is greeted by bubbling alpine creeks, smooth glaciated slabs, giant sequoias, deep dark-blue lakes, rock as far as the eye can see, meadows thick with a rainbow of flowers, alpine vistas, extensive conifer forests, shallow alpine tarns, domes, rivers, mining relics, cascades, pinnacled summits, and more.

This collection of attractions does not all exist in one location. The park covers nearly 1,200 square miles and ranges in altitude from below 3,000 feet along the Tuolumne and Merced River valleys to summits that top 13,000 feet. More than 800 miles of trail cut through the landscape, making a great number of hikes and diversity of landscapes accessible to anyone who wishes to park the car and explore the wilderness. Approximately a quarter of these trails are within 4 miles of a road, stretches that can be covered on a short day hike as defined in this book. This book includes 50 of my favorite excursions in and around Yosemite, chosen to introduce you to all of Yosemite's wonders. Although all are less than 8 miles round-trip, they range considerably in difficulty, length, and environment. I hope there are many that you find inviting.

1

ACCESSING YOSEMITE

Just 214 miles of roads cut lines across Yosemite's vast wilderness landscape. Five roads enter the park from the west: CA 140, CA 120, Evergreen Road, Cherry Lake Road, and CA 41, with only CA 120 extending across to the east end of Yosemite National Park. CA 140 follows the Merced River Canyon east from the town of Merced, past Mariposa and El Portal, and into Yosemite Valley. CA 120 climbs steeply out of the San Joaquin Valley, passing Groveland and approximately straddling the Tuolumne River–Merced River drainage divide as it enters Yosemite at Big Oak Flat and climbs to Crane Flat. At Crane Flat, the right-hand fork, Big Oak Flat Road, descends into Yosemite Valley, while CA 120, or Tioga Road, continues east to Tuolumne Meadows, Tioga Pass, and eventually Mono Lake. Evergreen Road is a spur off CA 120 that descends to Hetch Hetchy Reservoir just before the Big Oak Flat entrance station along CA 120. Cherry Lake Road is a second spur off CA 120; no walks from this destination are covered in this book, as the windy drive to Cherry Lake and nearby Lake Eleanor is lengthy. Similar scenery may be found at more easily accessible locations. And finally, CA 41 approaches Yosemite from the southeast, passing through Oakhurst and entering the park adjacent to Mariposa Grove and Wawona. It continues north, descending into the western end of Yosemite Valley. The only other spur of consequence is Glacier Point Road, forking from CA 41 at Chinquapin and traveling east to Glacier Point, always just a few miles from Yosemite Valley's southern rim. US 395 lies east of the park and connects to CA 120 in Lee Vining, 12 miles east of the Yosemite boundary at Tioga Pass.

Trailheads are of course confined to these roads, and the roads hence delineate the seven hiking regions covered in this guide: Hetch Hetchy Reservoir (accessed by Evergreen Road), Yosemite Valley (accessed by CA 140, CA 120, and CA 41), Glacier Point and Wawona (accessed by CA 41 and Glacier Point Road), Tioga Road and Tenaya Lake (along CA 120), Tuolumne Meadows (farther east along CA 120), Tioga Pass (the park's eastern boundary, accessed by CA 120), and Mono Lake and vicinity (east of Yosemite, accessed by CA 120 or US 395). Note that CA 120 east of Crane Flat and Glacier Point Road are closed November–May or beyond.

YOSEMITE'S SEASONS

Most people visit Yosemite in spring to see Yosemite Valley's raging waterfalls, or in summer, when school vacation permits a trip and temperatures are warmest. However, the lowest sections of the park, including Yosemite Valley, the Hetch Hetchy area, and Wawona, are accessible year-round and are snow-free during all but the coldest winter spells. Climbing just a few thousand feet brings you into the snowbelt, the mixed conifer zone, with snow cover generally from mid-November through March or April. Continued ascent into the montane, subalpine, and alpine reaches of the park, including passage along Tioga Road (CA 120) to Tuolumne Meadows and Tioga Pass, carries you to areas that are inaccessible for 7 months—from the first major snowfall in October or November until at least late May. Spring reaches the low elevations in April and the alpine in June. A warm, mostly dry summer follows. June–August is hot in Yosemite Valley, Wawona, and Hetch Hetchy and pleasant in Tuolumne Meadows and at Tioga Pass. By September, fall, with freezing nights, has arrived at the upper elevations, and within a month the yellow grass and coloring leaves have spread to Yosemite Valley. October brings the first snowfalls at the upper elevations, with snow already sticking in shadowed areas on the higher summits. Soon winter, with snow or persistent rain, has enveloped all of Yosemite. The plants, animals, and most visitors are again waiting for spring.

APPRECIATING THE PARK'S RICH NATURAL HISTORY

Every visitor to Yosemite will absorb some of the park's wonderful natural history—the granite walls and summits, as well as the multitude of plants and animals, that are experienced every time one steps out of the car and looks around. As you walk, take the time to look around you.

More than 400 species of mammals, birds, and reptiles call Yosemite home. Some of the species are seen by many park visitors: the ubiquitous California ground squirrels around Yosemite Valley and Glacier Point, inevitably begging for food; mule deer, frequently seen grazing in Yosemite Valley and Tuolumne Meadows; blue-and-black Steller's jays squawking as they fly from tree to tree; chipmunks and golden-mantled ground squirrels scurrying through the upper elevation forests; American black bears trotting confidently through the campgrounds at dusk, waiting for a camper to leave food unattended; marmots sunning themselves on high-elevation boulders; and many more.

Persistent searching—and a dose of luck—might lead to some treats: a weasel peering over a rock, a pika chirping from the middle of a high-elevation talus pile (or at Olmsted Point), a glimpse of a mountain lion in Yosemite Valley, or even a herd of Sierra bighorn sheep near Mono Pass. Other mammal species are so rare that they will likely go undetected during a lifetime of exploring the park. The Sierra Nevada red fox and the fisher are so rare that scientists generally see them only with motion-sensitive cameras. Animal species even continue to be found in Yosemite. In 2010 a new species, the Yosemite cave pseudoscorpion, was found lurking in granite talus in the park. Each species is found in a specific habitat—a particular elevation, meadows versus forests versus peaks—and only by hiking in many of Yosemite's habitats will a visitor have the opportunity to meet many of the park's permanent inhabitants.

In addition, 1,350 species of plants, from the giant stately sequoias to minute alpine cushion plants, have been recorded in Yosemite. Each species has its preferred habitat, delineated foremost by elevation (and therefore temperature) but also by moisture, soil depth, rock type, sunlight, and many more factors that create nearly infinite fine-scale habitats across a short distance—you will cross many on even a short walk.

In turn, plants inhabiting each so-called niche look different. At high elevations, savage winds and the heavy burden of a snowpack necessitate a short stature, while in a dense forest, being the tallest herb is advantageous because its leaves intercept the most sun. Plants in drier environments tend to have smaller leaves than those of their streamside compatriots. Meanwhile flowers come in all manner of shapes and colors, each long selected to maximize visitation by certain pollinators. A long tubular red flower attracts hummingbirds, while a wider, shorter, blue-tubed species will be visited by bees. Patchy, yet regular, wildfires are essential to create some habitats and therefore increase the diversity of species that exist in Yosemite. Some wildflowers and shrubs germinate only after an intense wildfire has cleared the overstory, while others thrive beneath a dark canopy of mature pines and even acquire energy directly from the trees' roots.

Although you may not be able to greet many plants by name, take the time to stare at the myriad of shapes and sizes, considering that no one species can live everywhere but that together plants do a remarkable job of exploiting every inhabitable inch of Yosemite. And of practical importance, two of the most colorful locations are meadows (especially those around 8,000 feet and in the alpine) and along stream banks.

The complex landscape of peaks, meadows, lakes, streams, and cliffs is the backdrop, the milieu that allows Yosemite's great biological diversity to exist. The geography owes its existence to the many different geologic processes that occurred over the last 100 million years. Here I introduce just three landmark geologic events and intertwined processes. The first is the creation of a vast block of granite, termed the Sierra Nevada batholith, between 105 and 85 million years ago. It formed deep underground as the

Pacific and North American tectonic plates collided, forcing the west-lying Pacific Plate deep into the earth. The plate melted, and some of the resultant magma erupted to form massive volcanoes, while the rest solidified underground to form the Sierra Nevada batholith. Today the volcanic rock has eroded and disappeared, while the granite is at the surface. The batholith is composed of many different variants of granite, each comprising its own distinctive combination of minerals and termed a pluton. Extensive planes of weakness exist within the rock, dating from its formation, and once the rock emerges on the Earth's surface, these weaknesses reveal themselves in several ways. First is exfoliation, whereby curved slabs of rock detach from the surface like the layers of an onion. Sentinel Dome and roadcuts along Tioga Road between Yosemite Creek and May Lake are excellent places to see this. Second are vast fractures that extend across the landscape, likely responsible for the general orientation of Yosemite Valley and many of its vertical walls, including the face of Half Dome.

The second set of geologic events includes various forces that caused the uplift of the Yosemite-area mountains and the surrounding Sierra Nevada. The timing and importance of different episodes of uplift are still uncertain, but geologists have established that a tall mountain range has existed in this location since the formation of the granitic batholith. The major river drainages and layout of the mountains have existed since this time. A more recent uplift event, beginning approximately 10 million years ago, led to a steepening of the mountain range. Hand in hand with uplift, and accentuated when uplift is greatest, is erosion, a slow but continuous process that breaks apart and moves rock from the highest summits toward sea level. Erosion occurs as water and ice flow over the rocks; as the rocks freeze and thaw each year, fracturing them; as animals (and now people) dislodge rocks; and in many other ways. Erosion is what has etched the major river valleys and shaped the peaks.

Third are repeated glaciations beginning just 2 million years ago. The glaciers scoured the landscape, scraping loose rock from the sides of valleys, shaping domes and summits, and polishing the rock. Glaciers did not create Yosemite Valley, but they steepened and smoothed its walls and scoured its base. In Tuolumne Meadows, all but the highest summits were submerged in the ice field, and today visitors can still feel the polished rock, visit endless beautiful lakes, and gaze at the pinnacled summits of the Cathedral Range—all the result of glacial action.

YOSEMITE'S HUMAN HISTORY

California Miwok Native Americans had inhabited Yosemite Valley for many centuries, probably millennia, before a party of explorers headed by Joseph Walker first looked down upon it in 1833. During the subsequent two decades, tensions between the European settlers and Native Americans in the Sierra Nevada foothills increased, leading to an offensive by the Mariposa Battalion in 1851. In search of the Ahwahneechee, the band of Miwok living in Yosemite Valley, these soldiers became the first Europeans to enter Yosemite Valley. This encounter ended badly for the Miwok, who were driven from their home. Just 4 years later the first tourist party reached the valley, and their drawings of Yosemite's waterfalls and vertical walls soon captivated the world. Yosemite quickly became another opportunity to earn easy money in the undeveloped West, as early settlers set up hotels and toll roads to extract money from the visitors streaming in.

Fortunately a few early visitors already recognized that this exquisite natural setting must be forever preserved and accessible to all—it must not be damaged by the extraction of its natural resources nor be allowed to fall into private ownership. Frederick Law Olmsted, a famed landscape architect, was one of its first advocates, successfully lobbying Congress to set aside Yosemite Valley and the Mariposa Grove of Big Trees for public use. President Abraham Lincoln signed the bill creating the Yosemite Grant in 1864, thus creating the first public park by action of the U.S. federal government. Galen Clark became Yosemite's first guardian, a quiet, respected man who was an effective caretaker in an era of ever-increasing visitation and divisive politics regarding how Yosemite should be managed and conserved.

John Muir, the man most associated with Yosemite, arrived a few years later. He spent the summer of 1869 in Yosemite's high country helping shepherd 2,000 sheep and quickly developed a boundless enthusiasm for Yosemite's landscape, geologic history, plants, and animals—as well as distaste for the damage to high meadows caused by sheep. His first attempts in 1881 to expand the Yosemite Grant to include the higher elevation reaches failed. For the following decade Yosemite's landscape became increasingly degraded by excessive tourism and construction in Yosemite Valley and vast flocks of sheep denuding its mountain meadows. In 1890 with the help of Robert Underwood Johnson, a friend and influential magazine editor, Muir succeeded in pushing the bill for an all-inclusive Yosemite National Park through Congress. It followed Yellowstone to become the United States' second national park.

Creating the national park was a veritable success, but Muir knew that a legislative designation was only the beginning. Next he needed to assemble a group of supporters to help expound the importance of undisturbed wilderness to a wider audience. The Sierra Club, founded in 1892, became his venue. It became and remains a powerful voice for both preservation of natural areas and the importance of people visiting these locations—for as John Muir knew well, the public will only become vested in a national park's worth as a place of national heritage if they experience the wonders for themselves. The same debate rages today, with policy makers debating the right balance between keeping Yosemite wild and natural and encouraging people to visit Yosemite, thereby becoming stronger proponents of its future. During your visit, consider how important the story of Yosemite National Park is to the history of the conservation movement and the existence of public lands—and that you as an engaged visitor are part of its future.

If you wish to learn more, exploring the nature and science sections of the park's website (**nps.gov/yose**) provides an excellent pre-visit introduction to Yosemite natural and human histories, while a trip to the Yosemite Valley Visitor Center, the Nature Center at Happy Isles, or the Pioneer Yosemite History Center in Wawona is a perfect way to begin your park visit. Many excellent books have also been written on its human and natural histories. Two of my favorites to read before your visit are *Geology Underfoot in Yosemite National Park* by Allen F. Glazner and Greg M. Stock and the out-of-print, but still available, history of Tuolumne Meadows, *Meadow in the Sky* by Elizabeth Stone O'Neill. *Flowering Shrubs of Yosemite and the Sierra Nevada* by Shirley Spencer and *Wildflowers of Yosemite* by Lynn Wilson, Jim Wilson, and Jeff Nicholas are excellent companions on the trail.

USING THIS BOOK

This book is written for everyone wanting to experience Yosemite's wonders on foot, whether you wish to take short excursions to the base of waterfalls or to vista points, moderate hikes to a grove of sequoias or to the summit of a granite dome, or more difficult adventures to the top of a peak or to the shores of an alpine lake. The walks range in length from 0.4 mile to 8 miles, with the majority in the always popular 2- to 5-mile range.

The description for each walk contains information on general trailhead location, trail use, distance and configuration, elevation range, facilities, hike highlights, a short overview, a detailed route description, and GPS coordinates (WGS84), as well as directions to the trailhead. The majority of hikes included are only accessible to hikers, although eight allow baby strollers on much of their length. Each hike lists the starting elevation and the elevation change, with cumulative elevation gained and lost given if there are significant undulations along the trail.

I have included several walks that are not on official trails, but all follow well-worn use trails, defined as a trail created by the passage of many feet. I recommend following these routes only if you have some prior hiking experience, such that you are confident you can distinguish the course of the trail from the surroundings. They generally lead to less-visited corners of Yosemite, but with that treat comes added responsibility: unconstructed trails are less resistant to erosion, making them poor choices just after snowmelt or heavy rain, when they are likely wet and muddy and easily damaged.

SELECTING A HIKE

Whether you are a new visitor to Yosemite or wishing to explore a new corner of the park, it can be a challenge to select the hike that best fits your expectations. This will be especially so because there is no single best hike to which I can direct you—my enthusiasm extends to every corner of Yosemite. Instead read the list of "Very Best Hikes" on pages ix–xi or peruse the chart on pages 220–222. I hope that this list and chart will let you pick a destination that perfectly matches your mood on a given day. And consider the following:

◪ Most walks in Yosemite Valley are crowded, for you are not the only person to have heard that it is beautiful. It is easy to be turned off by crowds, but remember that everyone is here for a good reason—the location really is spectacular. The Mariposa Grove near Wawona is similarly busy during the summer. If crowds of people take away from your enjoyment, visit in fall or winter, midweek, or early in the morning. I am always pleasantly surprised by how few people are on the trails before 10 a.m.

◪ Every walk included can be beautiful and rewarding, but some walks are most engaging during only part of the year. For instance, without flowers, the mid-elevation areas, such as near White Wolf, are less inspiring to me.

◪ No description given is intended to be a euphemism for boring—if a phrase such as "quiet forest walk" strikes you as such, pick a phrase that better matches your persuasions.

◪ The effort and time required to complete a given trail distance can vary enormously. Elevation (that is, low versus high), amount of elevation change, and trail condition all greatly affect your travel speed. In the high elevation regions around Tuolumne Meadows and Tioga Pass, you will walk more slowly than in Yosemite Valley, for there is less oxygen to breathe at the higher elevations. Use trails tend to be slower to walk than constructed trails, for they are narrower and often steeper. Consider, for instance, that the distance from White Wolf to Lukens Lake is nearly identical to the Twenty Lakes Basin circuit, but the latter will likely take twice as long.

WALKING WITH KIDS

The hike descriptions and recommendations are written with special consideration to families who are searching for the best walks to do with children. The introductory section for each of the seven regions highlights the hikes that are best suited to children. In this age of media entertainment and nonstop screens, it is incredibly important to introduce children to the outdoors at a young age. Most children love poking around nature, watching squirrels, finding a bird feather, collecting flowers, and jumping off rocks. Convincing them to hike (and simultaneously to leave Yosemite's natural treasures unpicked) is a little more difficult, but with some forethought, perfectly doable.

If your children balk at the idea of hiking, here are a few things to remember and some games that friends and I have been successful playing:

- Kids love rocks, including slabs, so pick a walk where they can enjoy a little rock walking.

- Before your walk, take your child to pick up a Junior Ranger booklet and pick an activity to do on the trail, so s/he can feel important as you walk.

- Remind your child that whoever walks steadily in front and is quietest will see the most animals.

- If you know a little about the trees or flowers, share it with your children, for they readily absorb natural history facts and are so proud about what they have learned. Have them count bundles of pine needles to differentiate between species or find flowers of all colors of the rainbow (just don't pick them).

- Make children feel proud of their walking abilities. Let children know in advance if you are going on a long walk and tell them that they are very capable of being able to complete it. I rate walks for my 5-year-old daughter by age, not miles, and she proudly rises to the occasion when she realizes that she gets to go on a hike rated above her age.

- Pick a destination with water play.

- Play hide-and-seek along the trail.

- Take walks with other children. Or make it a special occasion to have a one-on-one conversation with your child, instead of interacting only with the adults present.

- When the little legs begin to lag, have one adult go a few steps ahead and hide an occasional snack for a treasure hunt.

And don't be too hard on them:

◘ Remember that kids are more adversely affected by heat than adults are. Make sure that they wear wide-brimmed hats, drink plenty of water, eat food, and get lots of shady breaks.

◘ A very buggy trip will be a negative memory for a long time. During June and July avoid walks described as mosquito-prone.

◘ Promise a treat at the end of the day or trip—a special snack or a Yosemite-themed book at the visitor center.

STAYING SAFE

There is no reason to worry about your safety in a wilderness setting, but you must remember both to take care of your body's needs and to be aware of dangers that could arise. Cell phone reception is rare, and you may be alone on the trail, meaning that your party is responsible for getting yourselves safely back to the trailhead or fetching help if an injury occurs. If you are lost, especially off the trail, stay put. Members of your party or rescuers will find you more quickly if you haven't wandered farther afield.

Taking care of yourself: While exercising, you need to eat, drink, and maintain the correct body temperature to keep your body functioning. When on a hike, this requires a little forethought. Always wear sunscreen and a wide-brimmed hat. If you plan to be away from the car for more than 20 minutes, you should carry water, food, extra clothing (when appropriate), a map, and a small first-aid kit. It is important to drink water and eat as you exert yourself. Stop at least every 30 minutes for a drink and every 1–2 hours for a snack. For hikes up to 3 miles, carry a quart of water per person, and for longer excursions carry 2 quarts per person. In summer I include a jacket in my backpack when above 8,000 feet, where winds are stronger and thunderstorms more likely to build. During spring and fall I carry a warmer layer at all elevations. The tiniest of first-aid kits can simply contain a mild pain reliever (such as aspirin or acetaminophen), a few Band-Aids and larger bandages to cover a wound, and a roll of sports tape to hold bandages in place or cover a developing blister. Mosquito repellent is often an appreciated addition to your luggage, especially at the higher elevations in June and July and in Yosemite Valley in spring.

Avoiding dangers: During the spring, summer, and fall months, Yosemite is a fairly benign location, with mostly pleasant weather. However, there are environmental hazards of which you should be aware. Most injuries to park visitors occur because visitors ignore or are not familiar with warning messages issued by Mother Nature. Below is a brief overview on how to avoid common dangers.

CLIFFS AND WATERFALLS   Cliffs and steep granite slabs occur throughout Yosemite, including along many of the trails described in this book. There is nothing inherently dangerous about any of the hikes described, but poor judgment can take you too close to an escarpment. There are many drop-offs and unfenced (or poorly fenced) vista points, so don't clown around near an edge. Don't step forward or backward while staring through a camera viewfinder (or at a camera screen). And if you feel uneasy about the terrain you are on, turn around.

The tops of waterfalls require special attention, for the water-polished rock upstream of a waterfall is exceptionally slick, even when dry. People have slipped on this rock and slid into the watercourse and over the edge. Many have swum in the water upstream of the falls, been caught by an unexpectedly strong current, and been pulled over the falls. For this reason Emerald Pool, at the top of Vernal Fall, was closed to swimmers in the 1990s.

ALTITUDE SICKNESS   The walks around Tuolumne Meadows and Tioga Pass are at quite high elevations, and the air's oxygen content is considerably lower than at sea level. People not accustomed to high elevation are susceptible to altitude sickness. The best way to avoid it is to drink plenty of water, eat food, and walk slowly. Mild altitude sickness presents itself as a headache and a generally unwell feeling. With these symptoms it is safe to slowly continue to your destination. However, you should retreat to lower elevations if nausea persists or you feel that you are having an intensely difficult time breathing.

LIGHTNING   Thunderstorms are a regular summer occurrence around Tenaya Lake, Tuolumne Meadows, and Tioga Pass. If it is going to be a stormy day, clouds will begin to build up in the late morning or early afternoon, leading to mid- to late afternoon rain, hail, and lightning. You should avoid all open, exposed landscape, especially summits and exposed slabs, once you see the tall, dark thunderheads building. The sky can quickly transition from scattered clouds to a vicious storm. If you find yourself in an exposed location when the storm begins, stay out of shallow caves and away from overhangs. Then get in the lightning position, both to reduce the likelihood of a direct strike and to reduce the seriousness of any injury you may sustain. The National Outdoor Leadership School recommends squatting or sitting as low as possible, on a pile of clothes, and wrapping your arms around your legs. This position minimizes the chance of a ground current flowing through you. Close your eyes and keep your feet together to prevent the current from flowing in one foot and out the other.

STREAM CROSSINGS   Of the walks described here, 14 have a stream crossing without a constructed bridge. Many of these are trivial to hop across, but several require balancing on a log or rocks, a long leap, or wet feet. What can be trivial for most of the year can be frightening and dangerous during the week of peak flow, generally in June or early July. As you approach a crossing, keep your eyes alert to spur trails, indicating the most-used crossing point, often a downed log that is slightly upstream or downstream of the trail. If nothing is immediately obvious, take a few minutes to hunt for a safe, dry crossing before jumping into the water. If you must wade a river, find a sturdy stick or hiking pole, or join arms with a hiking partner to help maintain your balance. Bare feet are OK for a sandy river bottom, but keep your shoes on if it is rocky; you are much more likely to slip if your feet are uncomfortable and you lack a firm stance. When water flows are high, expect wet feet en route to Lukens Lake (Hike 24) and Mono Pass (Hike 38). It is inadvisable to ever enter a swiftly flowing large stream, including the Merced River in Yosemite Valley, when in flood or at high flow.

RATTLESNAKES   Western rattlesnakes, venomous vipers, are common up to elevations of 8,000 feet, although they can be found as high as 11,000 feet in midsummer. A triangular head; a regular pattern of beige, brown, and black splotches on their back; and a tail of rattles identify the species. That said, do not pick up any snakes, as rattlesnakes can vary considerably in color and young individuals do not yet have rattles. These rattlesnakes are not aggressive and give the characteristic tail shake—or rattle—to alert you to their presence. However, they will bite if threatened and when curled have a strike range of several feet. Note that most snakebites occur to people handling the snake or to rock climbers unknowingly placing a hand on a snake-containing ledge.

DEER AND BEARS   It is natural to be a little intimidated by Yosemite's black bears, but they have caused no fatalities and few injuries in Yosemite. All they want is your food. Be sure to store unattended food in bear lockers and keep your lunch and snacks with you at all times. If a bear does get hold of your food, it is hers; don't try to reclaim ownership of it. On the other hand, the seemingly harmless deer have actually caused several fatalities because people are more likely to attempt to retrieve stolen food from a deer. Heed the advice of signs throughout the park: don't approach or feed wildlife. Note that all bears in Yosemite are American black bears, but they range in color from light brown to black.

WATERBORNE ILLNESS   Water in Yosemite's streams and lakes may be contaminated with the protozoa *Giardia, Cryptosporidium,* or with various disease-causing bacteria. Although these contaminants are rare, it is advised that you do not drink untreated water, and instead fill your water containers from taps around the park. The closest water taps to each trailhead are indicated in the trail descriptions.

WINTER WEATHER   From November–April, and sometimes even until June, the high-elevation reaches of Yosemite are subjected to strong winter storms, dumping many feet of snow in 24 hours. The roads accessing these regions are closed in winter, so you will not experience quite these conditions. However, the same fronts pass through Yosemite Valley and Wawona, with the colder storms dropping snow and the others drenching rain. During these months, be sure to read the forecast. Unless you have excellent raingear and a heightened sense of adventure, it is best to venture no farther than the well-trodden tracks to Bridalveil Falls or to Lower Yosemite Falls on particularly stormy days.

LEAVE NO TRACE

Yosemite National Park is a national treasure and needs to be left the way you found it—leave only footprints and take only photographs, as the saying goes. You have likely chosen to visit Yosemite so you can unwind from daily life in a spectacular natural setting with limited signs of human visitation, and the next hiker wants to do exactly the same thing.

Most simply, leave no trace means that you take away all your trash, including toilet paper. Human garbage is the ugliest of sights in a wilderness area. But the phrase means more.

Leave no trace means:

- Leave the flowers attached to their roots. Nothing is sadder than watching a person yank off a woody stalk of rose spirea from atop Lembert Dome, clearly unaware of how long that branch took to grow, or seeing someone collect an enormous bouquet, only to cast it aside an hour later when it inevitably starts to wilt.

- Leave the rocks and pinecones for the next person to look at and enjoy. Let your child carry them for 5 minutes, but then place them back on the ground.

- Don't create new trails or widen existing trails, even if this means getting your feet wet when the trail is boggy.

- Decide not to follow use trails, even those described in this book, when they are boggy to avoid creating deep troughs. Constructed trails are hardier under these conditions.

- Keep wildlife wild by not feeding squirrels, birds, or other creatures.

- And my pet peeve: Don't collect all the rocks in a meadow and launch them into the nearby lake for fun, as this destroys animals' homes and exposes the roots of meadow plants, potentially killing them.

As for that toilet paper, bring a small zip-top bag to carry your used supplies and drop it in a garbage can at the end of the day. If your walk is long enough to require a toilet pit, carry a small plastic trowel and dig a 6-inch hole at least 100 feet from trails and water.

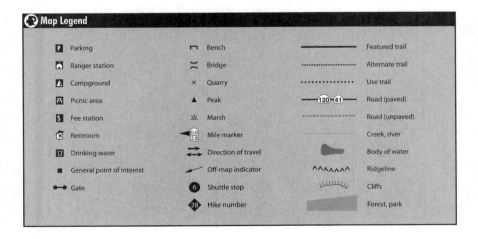

Map Legend

P Parking	Bench	————	Featured trail
Ranger station	Bridge	··············	Alternate trail
Campground	× Quarry	••••••••••	Use trail
Picnic area	▲ Peak	120–41	Road (paved)
S Fee station	Marsh	– – – – –	Road (unpaved)
Restroom	Mile marker	————	Creek, river
Drinking water	Direction of travel		Body of water
■ General point of interest	Off-map indicator	∧∧∧∧∧∧	Ridgeline
•—• Gate	6 Shuttle stop	⊔⊔⊔⊔⊔	Cliffs
	28 Hike number		Forest, park

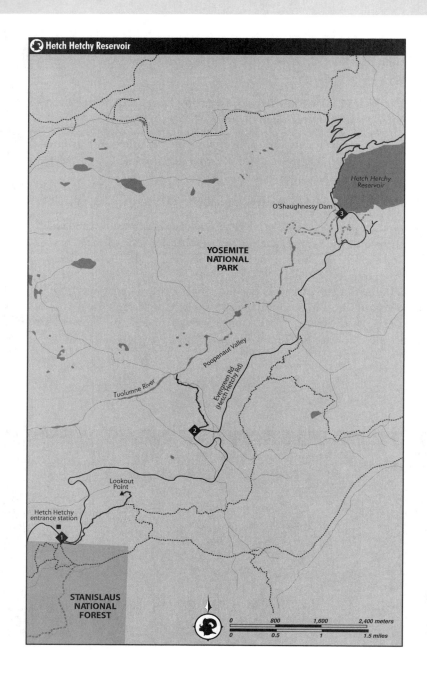

Hetch Hetchy
Reservoir

O'Shaughnessy Dam

YOSEMITE
NATIONAL
PARK

Poopenaut Valley

Evergreen Rd
(Hetch Hetchy Rd)

Tuolumne River

Lookout
Point

Hetch Hetchy
entrance station

STANISLAUS
NATIONAL
FOREST

0   800   1,600   2,400 meters
0   0.5   1   1.5 miles

HETCH HETCHY RESERVOIR

Regional Overview

Hetch Hetchy Reservoir is a symbol of the exploitation of a national park landmark, as well as an aspiration that the construction of the O'Shaughnessy Dam was the last time that one of our national treasures is so compromised. Sad as I am not to see Hetch Hetchy Valley as John Muir once did, this is still a location to visit. The bottom 312 feet of the valley are hidden, but the impressive granite walls rise an additional 2,000 feet, and the enormous body of dark-blue water provides a picturesque foreground. If you have never visited Hetch Hetchy, I strongly encourage you to take the walk to Wapama Falls (Hike 3).

The Hetch Hetchy region has a quite different atmosphere from the rest of Yosemite. There is the wonderful feel of continuous granite slabs and domes that dominates northern Yosemite, just with shorter summits; granite outcrops interspersed with drought-tolerant trees and shrubs are everywhere.

The three walks in this section are best done fall through spring, as they are all at low elevation and summer temperatures are sizzling. Lookout Point (Hike 1) is the easiest walk here for younger children, for Poopenaut Valley (Hike 2) includes a steep climb, and Wapama Falls (Hike 3) is a bit long. However, an energetic 8-year-old child would thoroughly enjoy Wapama Falls. Poopenaut Valley is a scenic location and reaching it is a lovely walk, but it is tough, so head there only if your knees and legs request a workout.

◻ ◻ ◻

1 Lookout Point

Trailhead Location: Hetch Hetchy entrance station

Trail Use: Hiking

Distance & Configuration: 2.8-mile out-and-back

Elevation Range: 4,750 feet at the start, with 560 feet of ascent/ descent

Facilities: A water faucet is located to the side of the buildings just to the right of the entrance station, but no toilet is at the trailhead.

Highlights: Fall colors, views to Hetch Hetchy, and a feel for the foothills

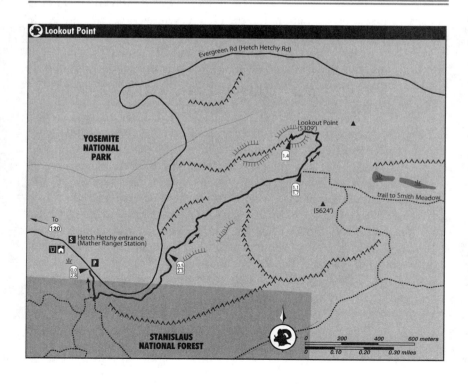

DESCRIPTION

This short hike leads to the summit of a small granite dome from which you can view Hetch Hetchy Reservoir and its surroundings—one of the few at this elevation that provides an expansive vista. Take the walk in the late afternoon for the best lighting. Also wonderful are the fall colors: the orange oak leaves and tall yellow grass.

THE ROUTE

Departing from the southern edge of the ranger's compound, locate a small trail disappearing south into a stand of tall incense cedars and Jeffrey pines. Just beyond is an unmarked X-junction where you turn left; straight ahead leads to Lookout Point by a much longer route. Heading left, you now parallel a broad turn in the Hetch Hetchy Road—a little frustrating to watch the cars as you walk, but there is no parking where the trail finally diverges from the road **(0.5 mile from start)**.

The trail switchbacks up a slope that was burned once about 20 years ago, and sections again in 2008; tall black snags dot the landscape, intermingled with black oak trees that escaped. A small stream flows through here in spring, providing moisture for an excellent wildflower display. In fall it is a landscape of tall yellow grass, seed heads, and coloring oak trees.

Where the slope ends, you enter a nearly flat and quite lush valley. The narrow trail continues between burnt trees. Ferns, tall scrubs, and seedlings thrive, all growing rapidly with the forest canopy removed. Soon you reach a T-junction **(1.1 miles)**, where the trail straight ahead leads to Hetch Hetchy Reservoir, while you take the left-hand fork

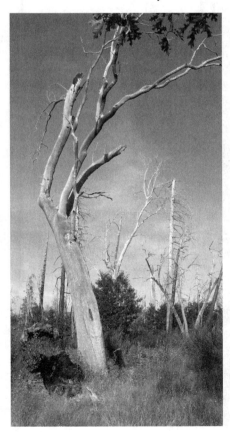
A partially burned oak tree

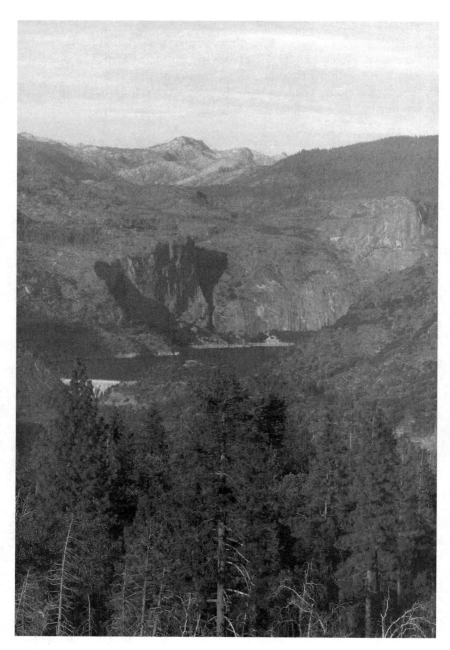

View to Hetch Hetchy Reservoir from Lookout Point

to climb up Lookout Point. The trail leads first north and then west to ascend the northern side of the small granite dome **(1.4 miles)**. Like so many of Yosemite's domes, a beautiful stunted Jeffrey pine emerges from a crack on the summit.

From the summit, especially with late-afternoon lighting, you will be treated to an aerial view of Hetch Hetchy Reservoir and the granite peaks to the north, a view usually obtained only by climbing difficult-to-reach summits such as Kolana Rock. In spring Tueeulala and Wapama falls will be obvious white streaks on the rock face. It is also simply a nice summit from which to take in the topography and vegetation of low-elevation western Yosemite, for there are few locations with views in this part of the park. When you have finished gazing about, return to your car the way you came **(2.8 miles)**.

TO THE TRAILHEAD
GPS Coordinates: N37° 53.592'   W119° 50.478'
Turn north from CA 120 onto Evergreen Road. This junction is located 1.1 miles west of the Yosemite entrance station at Big Oak Flat and 22.5 miles east of Groveland. (Note the sign with the current schedule for Hetch Hetchy day-use hours to avoid waiting behind a closed gate 15 minutes down the road.) After winding along Evergreen Road for 7.2 miles, you reach a T-junction with Hetch Hetchy Road. Turn right (east) and drive past Camp Mather, beneath a tall gateway, and past a gate that is locked each night. Beyond the T-junction, 1.3 miles later, you reach the Hetch Hetchy entrance station; here you are required to register your car. Park your car by the side of the road just beyond the entrance station and begin your walk on the southeastern side of the road.

2 Poopenaut Valley

Trailhead Location: Hetch Hetchy Road

Trail Use: Hiking

Distance & Configuration: 2.4-mile out-and-back

Elevation Range: 4,595 feet at the start, with 1,280 feet of descent/ ascent

Facilities: No facilities are at this trailhead, so be sure to fill your water bottles at the entrance station. Water and toilets are located at Hetch Hetchy Reservoir, an additional 4 miles down the road.

Highlights: Solitude, sandy banks and chilly swimming holes, and a steep climb

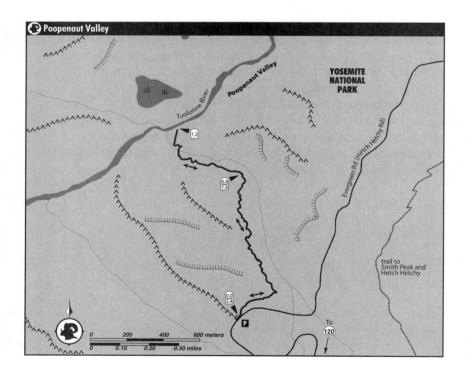

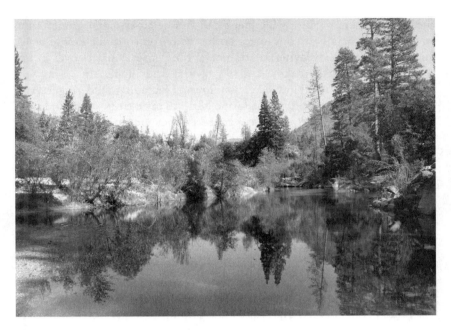

Tuolumne River in Poopenaut Valley

DESCRIPTION

This often-overlooked trail provides a beautiful, albeit steep, introduction to lower-elevation Yosemite. Best suited to the cooler months, the trail leads down a steep forested trail to the Tuolumne River. In fall you can enjoy beautiful beaches and swimming holes, and in spring enjoy the river's swirling waters. Visit this location mid-fall through spring but not summer, when temperatures are sizzling.

THE ROUTE

From the pullout, cross the street and head down a dry slope, colored by wildflowers in spring and parched in fall. After a brief traverse to the right, the trail enters cool forest cover. You are beneath a canopy of incense cedars and Douglas firs and beside a cascading creek. The sheltered draw that the trail follows contrasts sharply with the dry scrubby slopes you drove past along Hetch Hetchy Road.

This trail has not been updated, a nice way to note that it has not been regraded in recent decades. Instead, it drops at an approximate rate of 1,000 feet in 1 mile, twice as steeply as most switchbacking trails in the Sierra. There are a few big steps and simply a persistent grade. Take your time, especially if your knees bother you. You continue down, never far from the creek, weaving in and out of the denser conifer cover in the riparian zone and the oaks that grow on the drier slopes. In spring you will find some beautiful low-elevation flowers, including wild ginger. And suddenly the trail abruptly turns to the left **(0.8 mile from start)** and then flattens, indicating that you have reached Poopenaut Valley.

You now approach a large meadow, through which the creek you were following forms a deep channel. As you enter the opening, the trail peters out. USGS topo maps indicate that it continues along the western meadow edge to the riverbank, but equally obvious tracks cut across the meadow. In spring, when the ground will be marshy, you will select the left-hand option, both to stay dry and avoid damaging the meadow. In fall and winter, all choices are acceptable and walking through the tall, dry grass is appealing. Either way, you will shortly reach the river's edge. In spring you will be met by a raging torrent, while late season you will find delightful sandbanks for a picnic and a quiet river for swimming **(1.2 miles)**. But the water will be cold, for it is released from the chilly depths of Hetch Hetchy Reservoir a few miles upstream. Faint use trails that head upstream along the bank are animal tracks that rapidly become difficult to discern—do not be tempted to follow them. Return to your car the way you descended, taking your time and drinking plenty of water **(2.4 miles)**.

TO THE TRAILHEAD

GPS Coordinates: N37° 54.614'   W119° 48.877'

Turn north from CA 120 onto Evergreen Road. This junction is located 1.1 miles west of the Yosemite entrance station at Big Oak Flat and 22.5 miles east of Groveland. (Note the sign with the current schedule for Hetch Hetchy day-use hours to avoid waiting behind a closed gate 15 minutes down the road.) After winding along Evergreen Road for 7.2 miles, you reach a T-junction with Hetch Hetchy Road. Turn right (east) and drive past Camp Mather, beneath a tall gateway, and past a gate that is locked each night. Beyond the T-junction, 1.3 miles later, you reach the Hetch Hetchy entrance station; here you are required to register your car. Continue along Hetch Hetchy Road for another 3.9 miles. As you complete a large curve, keep your eyes open for a small turnout on the right side of the road and a metal sign on the left side of the road indicating the start of the trail to Poopenaut Valley.

3 Wapama Falls

Trailhead Location: Hetch Hetchy Reservoir

Trail Use: Hiking

Distance & Configuration: 4.8-mile out-and-back

Elevation Range: 3,813 feet at the start, with a cumulative elevation change of ±600 feet

Facilities: Water and toilets are not located at the trailhead but instead along the road 0.3 mile before the dam. Stop briefly at a small parking area after a series of ranger cabins. Water and toilets are also present at the entrance to the backpacker campground, farther along the one-way loop road. There is even a drinking fountain on the dam.

Highlights: Impressive rock walls and body of water, as well as Kolana Rock's striking form

DESCRIPTION

The nearly level walk to Wapama Falls is especially rewarding in spring, when the path is lined with wildflowers and Tueeulala and Wapama falls drench the trail. Year-round it is a scenic walk above the banks of Hetch Hetchy Reservoir.

THE ROUTE

From the parking area, descend alongside the road to the dam. Turn left and cross the O'Shaughnessy Dam, stopping to read the excellent information placards and enjoy the view. The steep dome overshadowing the right shore of Hetch Hetchy Reservoir is Kolana Rock. The gushes of water cascading down Wapama Falls to the east and the smaller Tueeulala Falls to the west (left) are impossible to miss in spring, while in fall Tueeulala will certainly be dry and Wapama Falls a distant trickle. Staring at the steep walls and narrow body of water is of course an unnatural vista, and as much as I wish that I were able to descend into Hetch Hetchy Valley as John Muir did, I find that the dark-blue reservoir and granite walls are a beautiful panorama.

Once across the dam, you enter a tunnel, which cuts through an otherwise impassable cliff. It has recently been updated with new lighting

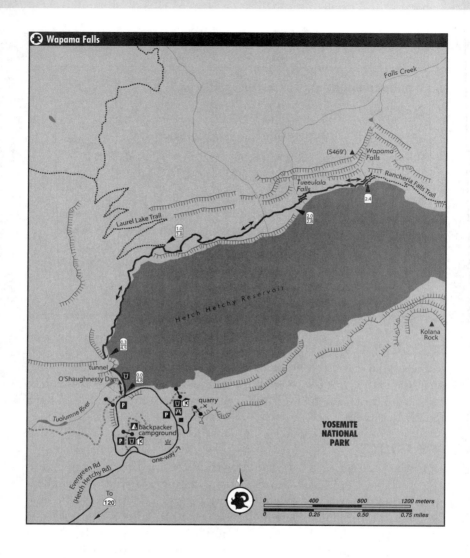

and a flatter floor. Beyond the tunnel **(0.3 mile from start),** you are on an old road, created during the construction of the dam. When full, the water will be just a few feet below the trail, but this is a rare occurrence, and you will almost always see the bare, bleached talus piles that form a bathtub ring around the reservoir.

You begin your walk beneath live oaks, manzanitas, and bay laurel trees. Poison oak is abundant at the perimeters, but the trail is plenty wide here to avoid it. Wildflowers, including harlequin lupines, color the path's edges in spring. Note one location where a recent rockfall has cleared a strip of vegetation above the trail and sent boulders tumbling onto the trail. Gaining little elevation, you continue along the pleasant trail to a junction where the left-hand branch climbs to Laurel Lake and Lake Vernon, while you turn right on the trail to Wapama Falls and beyond to Rancheria Falls **(1.0 mile)**.

Bearing right, you alternatively cross open slabs and pass small patches of meadow growing in an incredibly thin soil layer. In spring water pools on the underlying rock, creating miniature wetlands with beautiful flower displays, while by summer the soil and vegetation are parched. The few trees present, manzanitas and foothill pines, undoubtedly have their roots in cracks in the rock, accessing deeper, moister soil.

Soon you cross an unnamed seasonal tributary, whose waters cascade down the broken cliffs above and often straight over the trail. Beyond, the flat slabs transition into a steeper slope. For the next 3 miles, the trail follows a ledge system, a corridor through the otherwise impassable slabs. Shortly you cross the base of Tueeulala Falls on a wooden footbridge **(2.0**

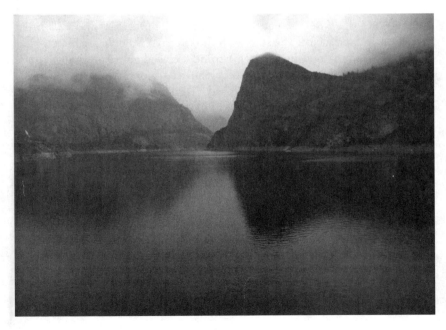

Kolana Rock overlooking Hetch Hetchy Reservoir

miles); this waterfall flows only during peak runoff, for it is actually a branch of Falls Creek (the Wapama Falls creek) that fills only during the highest water conditions. (USGS topo maps mark Tueeulala Falls at the location of the previous tributary.) Continuing along, you find yourself under dense forest cover in places and on open talus slopes elsewhere. Stretches of trail have been recently rebuilt, and you can savor the beautiful stonework on the path. A final short descent takes you to the five bridges that cross Falls Creek as it splays across a giant boulder fan at the base of Wapama Falls **(2.4 miles)**. In autumn you must cross the bridges to even see the waterfall, for the water actually cascades down the east-facing side of a corner. In spring you will be aware of the falls before you reach the bridges, for there will be a thundering sound and drenching spray. On one occasion in early June, water was flowing over the bridge and I was taking a shower until I was well beyond the bridges; take care under these conditions, for two people were recently swept off the bridge. Return to your car by the same route **(4.8 miles)**.

TO THE TRAILHEAD
GPS Coordinates: N37° 56.789'   W119° 47.257'
Turn north from CA 120 onto Evergreen Road. This junction is located 1.1 miles west of the Yosemite entrance station at Big Oak Flat and 22.5 miles east of Groveland. (Note the sign with the current schedule for Hetch Hetchy day-use hours to avoid waiting behind a closed gate 15 minutes down the road.) After winding along Evergreen Road for 7.2 miles, you reach a T-junction with Hetch Hetchy Road. Turn right (east) and drive past Camp Mather, beneath a tall gateway, and past a gate that is locked each night. Beyond the T-junction, 1.3 miles later, you reach the Hetch Hetchy entrance station; here you are required to register your car. Continue along Hetch Hetchy Road for another 7.9 miles, passing an expansive ranger and water company employee residence, a toilet, and the dam itself, before finding an elongated parking area along the right side of the road. Note that the last 0.5 mile of road is a one-way loop.

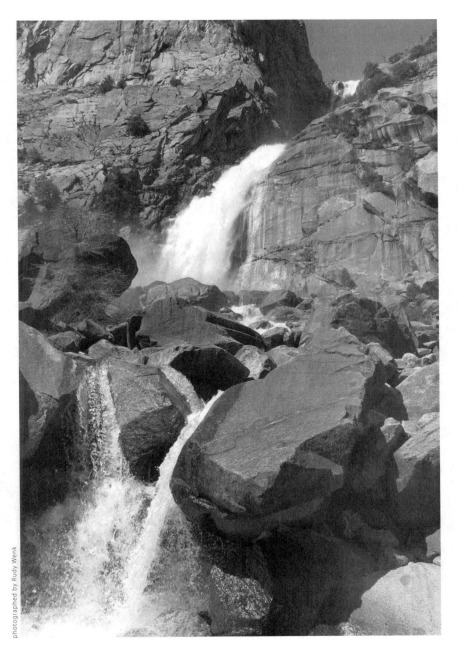

photographed by Rudy Wenk

Wapama Falls

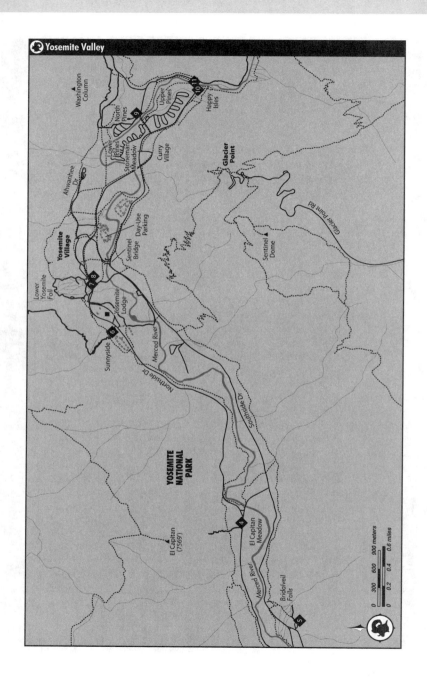

Yosemite Valley

YOSEMITE VALLEY

Regional Overview

The centerpiece of Yosemite National Park, Yosemite Valley absolutely lives up to its reputation as one of the more stunning settings on Earth. The 6 miles of valley floor are lined by 3,000-foot walls, pinnacles, and waterfalls. The iconic shapes of El Capitan and Half Dome dominate the skyline. At the valley's eastern end is Tenaya Canyon, with its even more expansive granite slabs reaching to the summit of taller peaks.

Because others share my admiration for Yosemite Valley, it is also very, very crowded, especially during late spring and summer months. This is not a location to visit if you seek solitude. But it is likewise not a place to shun just because you will not be by yourself. People visit iconic attractions because they are just so exquisite. The easiest way to avoid most of the people is to stay in the park and begin your walks early in the day; until 10 a.m. the crowds are manageable (and summer temperatures more pleasant). Fall is quieter, but of course the waterfalls are only dribbling and the flowers have faded. While the Yosemite Valley walks that climb upward are icy (and closed) in winter, the walks on the valley floor are accessible year-round, and a thin layer of snow is a beautiful decoration. May and early June are the best times to see the waterfalls roaring, and it is worth putting up with the crowds to visit then.

The walks climbing above the valley floor are all steep and not ideal for young children, but the valley floor walks (Bridalveil Falls, Base of El Capitan, Swinging Bridge and Superintendent's Bridge, Lower Yosemite Fall, and Mirror Lake) are short and have much less elevation change. The Base of Vernal Fall (Hike 10) is the first of the waterfall hikes to attempt as a family—and if your children are sufficiently engaged by the drenching

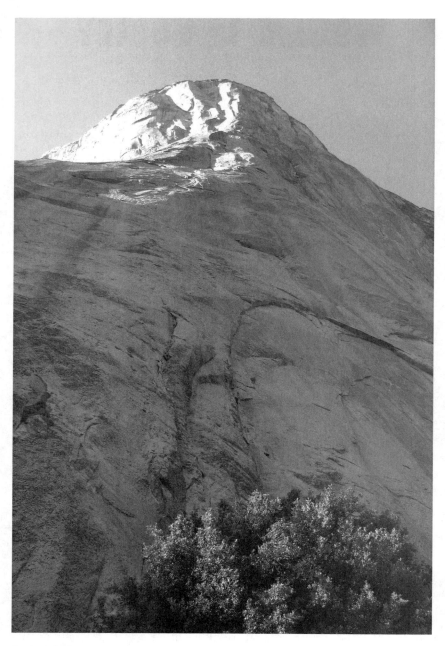

Staring 3,000 feet up the face of El Capitan (see page 34)

water, you may just find that they are willing to continue upward; kids seem to like the steep steps a lot more than adults. The two more difficult valley hikes, Upper Yosemite Fall (Hike 6) and Mist Trail and Clark Point (Hike 11) offer superb views of waterfalls and surrounding granite slabs and domes, but they are steep and longer—that is, difficult. Two hikes that finish in Yosemite Valley, the Panorama Trail and the Four Mile Trail, are described in the next section, Glacier Point Road and Wawona. I recommend them as one-way hikes from Glacier Point into the valley, allowing you to enjoy the stunning views obtained from the middle of the valley's walls without having to climb uphill.

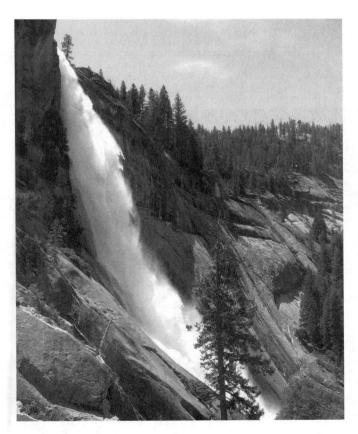

Nevada Fall from the Mist Trail (see page 63)

4 Base of El Capitan

Trailhead Location: El Capitan Meadow, west end of
Yosemite Valley

Trail Use: Hiking

Distance & Configuration: 0.8-mile out-and-back

Elevation Range: 3,970 feet at the start, with 280 feet of ascent/
descent

Facilities: No amenities are at the trailhead. The closest toilets
are at Bridalveil Falls, and toilets and water are available at
Yosemite Lodge.

Highlights: Surreal views of a 3,000-foot granite face

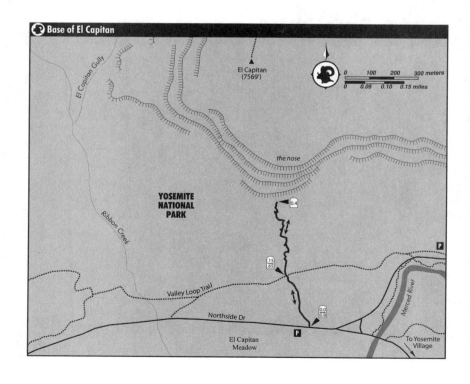

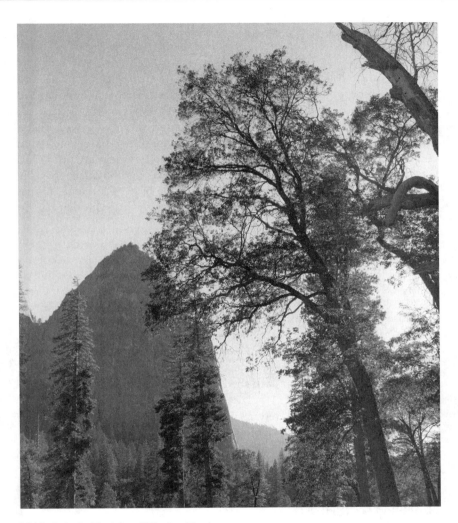

Middle Cathedral Rock from El Capitan Meadow

DESCRIPTION

The unmarked use trail to the base of El Capitan gives you an unusual panorama of the imposing granite face—straight up and up and up. From the base you lack the perspective gained from standing in a nearby meadow, making it difficult to estimate the wall's height. Combine this walk with a visit to El Capitan Meadow to admire the mountain from a bit farther back.

THE ROUTE

The unmarked, but obvious, trail begins at the far eastern end of El Capitan Meadow, about 300 feet after the two roads entering the meadow merge. Walking along the right-hand edge of an open black oak and ponderosa pine woodland, you reach a large opening through which the Valley Loop Trail passes **(0.15 mile from start)**. Walk north to the back of the opening—in the direction of El Capitan. Here you will find a use trail that zigzags quite steeply up to the monolith's base. The many climbers heading for the rock have created a well-worn route, allowing you to avoid burrowing into the dense manzanitas and huckleberry oaks that cover the slope. As you exit the scrub at the base of the rock, take a look at where you are—the start of the trail here is a little hidden on the return **(0.4 mile)**.

Now walk up to the base of El Cap and touch the nearly 3,000-foot wall. Without trees for scale, the wall feels dimensionless to me and I'd be hard pressed to decide if it were 100 or 10,000 feet high. Look up, up, up through binoculars if you have them, maybe glimpsing climbers high above you. You are standing just to the right of the most famous route, the Nose, which approximately follows the corner where the eastern and western halves of the face meet. Notice how few newly fallen rocks are at the base of the wall. Like most of Yosemite Valley, it is composed of very solid rock. The vegetated slope you just walked up is composed of rock from much older falls, so rock is indeed shed here as well, but by chance there has not been recent activity.

When you are finished, retrace your steps to the car **(0.8 mile)**. Before you drive away, walk into El Capitan Meadow, just across the road, to gain a second perspective on the peak and to enjoy some of the other walls and pinnacles gracing the western half of Yosemite Valley, including Cathedral Rocks and Cathedral Spires to the south.

TO THE TRAILHEAD

GPS Coordinates: N37° 43.452' W119° 38.071'

Two roads, Northside Drive and Southside Drive, run the length of Yosemite Valley. For most of their length they are both one-way, with traffic traveling east (toward Half Dome) on Southside Drive and west (out of the valley) on Northside Drive. El Capitan Meadow is accessed from Northside Drive. It lies 2.5 miles west of Yosemite Lodge, just beyond where a crossover road merges with Northside Drive.

5 | Bridalveil Falls

Trailhead Location: West end of Yosemite Valley

Trail Use: Hiking

Distance & Configuration: 0.8-mile out-and-back

Elevation Range: 3,970 feet at the start, with 100 feet of ascent/ descent

Facilities: Toilets are at the trailhead. Water is available at many locations around Yosemite Village, Yosemite Lodge, and Curry Village.

Highlights: Wonderful late-afternoon lighting, forever-moving stream of water, and year-round water

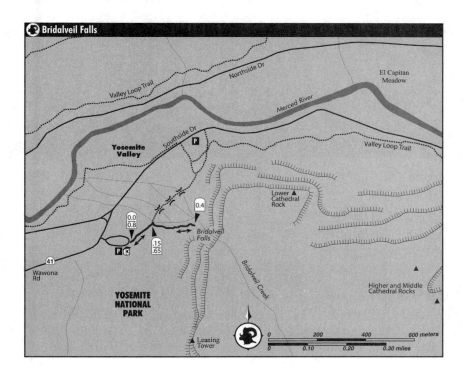

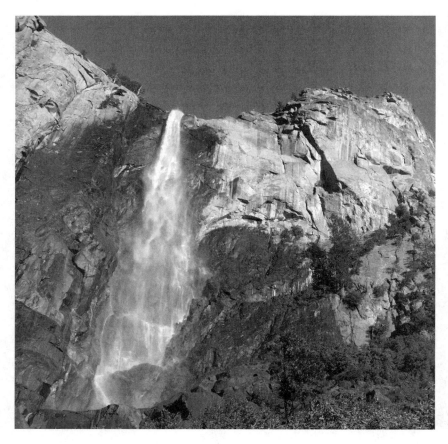

Bridalveil Falls

DESCRIPTION

The short walk to Bridalveil Falls is a must-do for every Yosemite tourist. The lighting is best in the late afternoon, beautifully illuminating the stream of water and U-shaped hanging valley at the top of the fall.

THE ROUTE

From the parking lot, head east on the wide paved trail. A little beyond the parking area, the track forks **(0.15 mile from start)**. Stay right; the left-hand track takes you to the El Capitan vista point along Southside Drive. Your trail climbs gently alongside one of the four boulder-filled channels that comprise Bridalveil Creek below the waterfall. As you approach the fall, the surrounding vegetation becomes lush, for the waterfall's year-round spray keeps the plants, including thickets of wild grapes, well watered.

Next you reach the falls themselves, with Bridalveil Creek plunging 620 feet over a vertical granite lip onto a steep pile of talus **(0.4 mile)**. The waterfall is shaded in the early morning but catches the afternoon light; beautiful rainbows are created, but they are as ephemeral as the wind is fickle, forever carrying the spray in a new direction. In spring the enormous flow masks the granite wall, while in fall the rock face shares center stage with the waterfall, two equally magical views of the location. To the right (southwest) of the fall is the overhanging wall of the Leaning Tower and to its left (east) the nearly as steep Cathedral Rocks. I have always been particularly attracted to the top of Bridalveil Falls, for unlike most of Yosemite Valley's waterfalls, there is no trail zigzagging to the top of the waterfall, giving the hanging valley above an aura of mystery.

Enjoy the waterfall from the large, rock wall–enclosed viewing area before retracing your steps to the car **(0.8 mile)**.

TO THE TRAILHEAD
GPS Coordinates: N37° 43.009' W119° 36.060'
Two roads, Northside Drive and Southside Drive, run the length of Yosemite Valley. For most of their length they are both one-way, with traffic traveling east (toward Half Dome) on Southside Drive and west (out of the valley) on Northside Drive. When entering Yosemite Valley on CA 120 (Big Oak Flat Road) or CA 140 (via El Portal), you enter the valley to the west of where the roads diverge and become one-way and you are funneled onto Southside Drive. When entering Yosemite Valley on CA 41 (from Wawona), you merge onto Southside Drive farther east. The Bridalveil Falls parking area is located on CA 41, just before it merges with Southside Drive. If you are on CA 41, the parking lot is on your right, 1.6 miles beyond the Wawona Tunnel. If you have come from CA 140 or CA 120, 0.9 mile after you turn onto the one-way road, you will see signs indicating that you should stay in the left lane for Yosemite Valley destinations and the right lane for Wawona and Bridalveil Falls. Turn right, as if you were heading out of the valley, and immediately turn left into the Bridalveil Falls parking area. Bridalveil Falls is not serviced by any of the free shuttle routes.

6 Upper Yosemite Fall

Trailhead Location: Yosemite Valley Shuttle stop 7, Sunnyside Campground (Camp 4)

Trail Use: Hiking

Distance & Configuration: 6.4-mile out-and-back

Elevation Range: 3,990 feet at the start, with a cumulative elevation change of ±3,300 feet

Facilities: Water and toilets are available in Camp 4. Just detour a short distance into the campground before beginning your walk.

Highlights: Climbing past a tall, gushing waterfall; Yosemite Valley views; and vertical rock walls

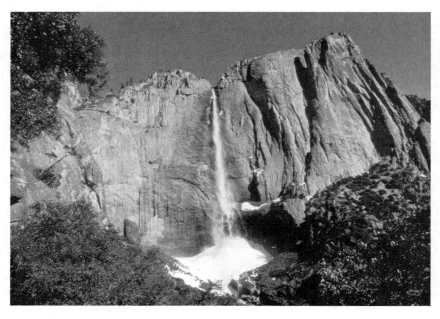

Upper Yosemite Fall in winter

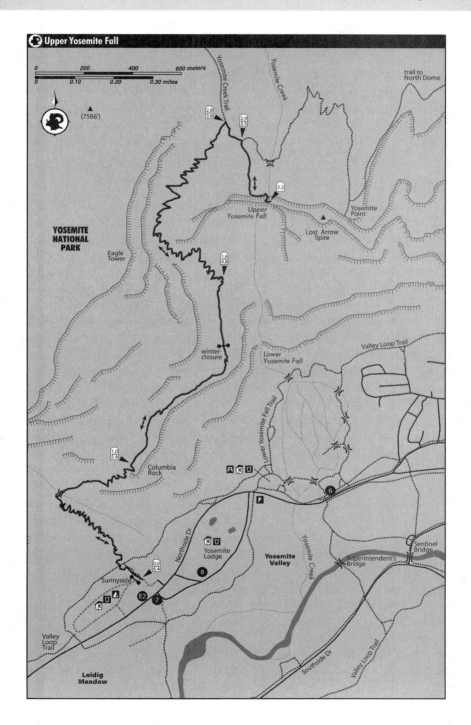

DESCRIPTION

This is an iconic Yosemite Valley walk, climbing alongside the vertical face down which the 1,430-foot Upper Yosemite Fall pours and then peering back down on the stream of water from a well-perched vista. As an added bonus, your views of Yosemite Valley and the Yosemite high country become more expansive and aerial with each step. This trail is accessible early spring through fall, but go in May and June for the most impressive water. Start your hike early in the day to avoid a hot climb.

THE ROUTE

Departing from the north end of the Camp 4 parking area, you jog briefly left onto the Valley Loop Trail and almost immediately back off it to the right. You then begin an endlessly switchbacking climb through a scrub oak forest. Large boulders lie scattered around, reminders of past rockfalls. Elegant rock walls support the short, even, but quite steep switchbacks, indicating the work that went into building the trail. Many tight corners later, you reach a shelf, basically a passageway in the steep terrain where the trail can head sideways. You cross a bridge and begin a long east-trending traverse toward the fall. Before long the traverse is broken by another cluster of switchbacks, directing the trail a little higher to avoid a cliff. Above is Columbia Rock **(1.0 mile from start)**, providing your first expansive vista to the southeast. From here you can see the steep summit of Mount Clark, a peak that will become ever more prominent as you climb higher. You also have magnificent views of Yosemite Valley, for you are now approaching the midpoint of its walls; it is from this stance that you feel most surrounded by the vertical walls. From the valley floor you are just looking up, from the valley rim you are looking down, but from the middle you are part of them. Sit, enjoy, and have a snack and water break.

Beyond Columbia Rock there are a few trees to shade you, which are welcome to hikers because this trail is south-facing and toasty by midmorning. The trail continues its traverse, then descends gently, makes two tight switchbacks, and turns left into the amphitheater holding Yosemite Falls. Here you are on a quite narrow ledge—indeed the route looks almost improbable from below—yet you will feel very secure as you hike.

Passing a gate, indicating where the trail may be officially closed in midwinter, you are now walking past rock boulders interspersed with scattered trees and beautiful wildflowers. Take the time to stare up at the steep rock face and across to Upper Yosemite Fall. In spring and early summer, all you will see is gushing water, obscuring the granite wall. In late summer and fall there will be only a trickle—or no water at all—and your eyes will be drawn to the intricacies of the rock face, beautiful water stains, and Lost Arrow Spire. If you are ascending in winter, you will be treated to the snow cone, a large pile of ice that accumulates at the base of the fall. The ice forms as the water falls through the cold air. (During much of winter you can ascend to this point on dry ground, but the set of switchbacks that climb next to Upper Yosemite Fall are likely to remain snowy until March or April.)

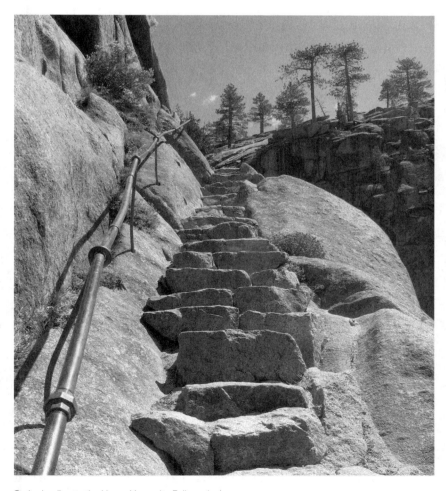

Stairs leading to the Upper Yosemite Fall overlook

At the end of this traverse you enter a stand of trees, including red-barked incense cedars and big-leaf maples, and the trail soon resumes its switchbacking climb **(1.6 miles)**. The zigzags maneuver you slowly to the northwest toward a passable gully in the otherwise vertical walls. You again leave tree cover behind and ascend a dry, gravelly slope, the path of Yosemite Creek before a glacial moraine pushed it into its current course. As you cross a small trickle of water, note a large open boulder pile to your east (right); this is one of the best photo locations, for trees do not obscure the view to Upper Yosemite Fall. If the wall is in the shade on your morning ascent, take your photo on the way down when the sun will be illuminating from the southwest.

You climb ever upward, likely feeling quite beat from the relentless grade and endless switchbacks. You are not alone, for this is a tough stretch of trail. The hard, gravelly ground is tough on your feet, the rock steps and ramps are often sand covered and slippery, and most days it is blazing hot. So stop, drink plenty of water, eat some food, and look up at the beautiful granite walls to remind you why you're here. Enjoy the shrubs that are your constant companions: chinquapins with golden-bottomed leaves and prickly fruit and red-barked manzanitas. A few tall Jeffrey pines and white firs indicate that you are approaching the rim, and indeed soon there are more trees, then a forest, flatter topography, and a trail junction. The trail up Yosemite Creek continues straight ahead, while you turn to the right, toward Yosemite Point and North Dome **(2.8 miles)**.

Ascending quickly to the crest of a sparsely forested ridge, you will note a use trail created by hikers that descends toward the lip of Upper Yosemite Fall **(2.9 miles)**. Follow the well-worn path past a weathered Jeffrey pine and then down the cliff face to look over the lip of the falls **(3.2 miles)**. At least you feel as though you are descending a cliff face, but handrailings and stone stairs are along the way, and safety rails ring the large viewing platform, so you needn't worry about your safety. But don't be foolish and swim in the pools above the falls or try and hang over the railings, for people do fall. (This vista is perfectly safe for adults, but I would hesitate to take a child, even a 10-year-old, to this location if they don't listen to your warnings.)

Returning to the main trail, retrace your steps to Yosemite Valley **(6.4 miles)**.

If you have time, energy, and water supplies remaining, I recommend continuing to Yosemite Point, an additional 1.8 miles round-trip and a location with even more panoramic views. To reach it, turn right (east) at the trail junction to the Yosemite Falls overlook, crossing Yosemite Creek on a wooden footbridge. Never, never swim, wade, or even walk on dry rock in this section of Yosemite Creek. The rock base is unbelievably polished, making it very easy to slip and continue over the falls. The trail switchbacks up an open slabby slope and then passes through a small stand of conifers. Just beyond is a metal sign pointing left to North Dome, while you stay straight ahead and reach the valley rim at Yosemite Point.

TO THE TRAILHEAD
GPS Coordinates: N37° 44.541' W119° 36.126'

Unless you are camping at Camp 4, no parking is available at this trailhead. A limited amount of parking is available at Yosemite Lodge, but it is recommended that you leave your car at your campsite, at the location of your other valley accommodation, or park at the large visitor parking lot at shuttle bus stop 1. To reach this parking lot, drive east (toward Half Dome) on Southside Drive until you reach a stop sign at Sentinel Bridge, 4.1 miles from where CA 41 merges with Southside Drive. At this stop sign, straight ahead takes you to Curry Village, while left across Sentinel Bridge leads to Yosemite Village and Yosemite Lodge. Turn left. After 0.3 mile you reach a second stop sign; turning left takes you to Yosemite Lodge, while you turn right to Yosemite Village. Continue east for 0.1 mile to another stop sign and turn right into a large dirt parking area. Park your car and wait for the shuttle bus. Get off at stop 7, Sunnyside Campground (Camp 4).

7 Lower Yosemite Fall

Trailhead Location: Yosemite Valley Shuttle stop 6, Lower Yosemite Fall

Trail Use: Hiking, stroller accessible

Distance & Configuration: 1.2-mile loop

Elevation Range: 3,970 feet at the start, with a cumulative elevation change of ±50 feet

Facilities: Toilets, water, and a picnic area are 0.1 mile from the start of the walk. Bicycle parking is available just east of the shuttle stop.

Highlights: Impressive view of Lower Yosemite Fall and braided creeks on a shaded stroll accessible to all

DESCRIPTION

A must-do hike for every visitor to Yosemite Valley, this walk takes you right to the base of Lower Yosemite Fall, thundering in spring and dry by late summer, when you gaze upon an impressive rock wall. The loop walk takes you across the many forks of Yosemite Creek en route to the fall.

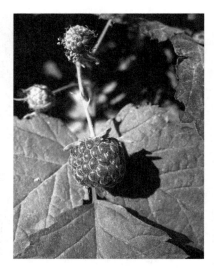

A wild raspberry

THE ROUTE

Beginning at shuttle stop 6, you walk 300 feet north to the main trail, turn left, and begin a clockwise loop along a paved trail. The endpoint of this walk is of course Lower Yosemite Fall, but the loop walk, constructed after the devastating January 1997 floods, embraces Yosemite Creek. After plummeting down the cliff face as a single thundering flow, Yosemite Creek hits the valley floor and transforms into a sluggish, braided creek. The walk takes you along and repeatedly across the many strands. Indeed, you now cross two bridges in rapid succession, the first across the main channel and then across a subsidiary flow, dry by midsummer. Passing a large complex of restrooms and a picnic area, the trail bends right (north) toward the waterfall (**0.2 mile from start**).

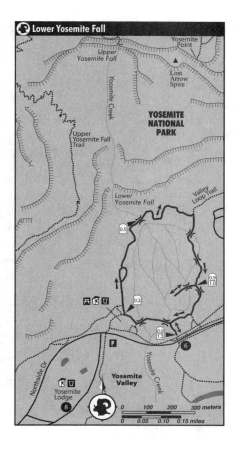

Continuing due north, take the time to enjoy the sculptures installed when the trail was refurbished. One shows the trail and surrounding landscape in beautiful detail. Another memorializes John Muir. Elsewhere beautiful granite plates are used as pavement around trees. You will of course also look straight ahead, for this stretch of trail is aligned to provide views of Upper, Middle, and Lower Yosemite falls. After a short climb through incense cedars and ponderosa pines, the trail bends right into a grove of live oaks and reaches the base of the falls (**0.5 mile**).

In spring the sound of the water will now be deafening and the spray rapidly drenches you, while by midsummer you will instead hear the sounds of children playing in the creek. The view also changes notably with the season. In winter there is usually a narrow stream of water and the surrounding rock is covered with ice, in spring the rock face is completely hidden behind the gushing water, and in late summer and autumn you will be admiring the steep rock face and its watermarks. When water levels are low, it is worth detouring onto the boulders in the creek for a better view and a sense of how effectively the water polishes rocks. But walk with care, as those smooth river boulders are very slippery—and do not leave the track when water levels are high. Note that the waterfall is best viewed in the middle of the day, for it is shaded in the early morning and again by midafternoon.

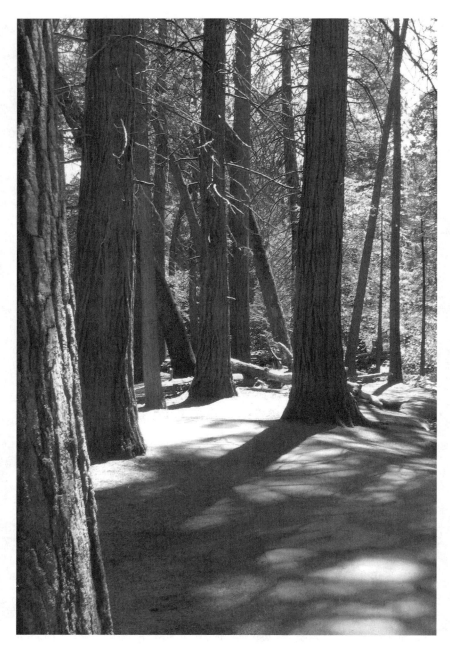

Ponderosa pines and incense cedars lining the trail

Continuing along, the trail now weaves around trees and boulders as it contours along the edge of the cliff face. At a T-junction you turn right, away from the waterfall, and begin your return to the shuttle stop; straight ahead the Valley Loop Trail continues east. Boulder-filled and often-dry creek beds lie to either side of you, and you cross one of them twice before reaching another junction **(0.9 mile)**. For a quick and worthwhile detour, take the right-hand spur trail across the bridge to a vista point. Here you can again see both waterfalls and with only trees—not people—as foreground. Retracing your steps to the main trail **(1.0 mile)**, continue along, admiring the expanses of ferns and thickets of tasty raspberries and thimbleberries. Stay right at the next junction and a little beyond take the left-hand spur trail, leading you back to the shuttle stop **(1.2 miles)**.

TO THE TRAILHEAD
GPS Coordinates: N37° 44.744' W119° 35.623'
No parking is available at this trailhead. A limited amount of parking is available at Yosemite Lodge, but it is recommended that you take the Yosemite Valley Shuttle to the trailhead. Leave your car at your campsite or valley accommodation, or park at the large visitor parking lot at shuttle bus stop 1. To reach this parking lot, drive east (toward Half Dome) on Southside Drive until you reach a stop sign at Sentinel Bridge, 4.1 miles from where CA 41 merges with Southside Drive. At this stop sign, straight ahead takes you to Curry Village, while left across Sentinel Bridge leads to Yosemite Village and Yosemite Lodge. Turn left. After 0.3 mile you reach a second stop sign; turning left takes you to Yosemite Lodge, while you turn right to Yosemite Village. Continue east for 0.1 mile to another stop sign and turn right into a large dirt parking area. Park your car and wait for the shuttle bus. Get off at stop 6, Lower Yosemite Fall.

8 Swinging Bridge and Superintendent's Bridge

Trailhead Location: Yosemite Valley Shuttle stop 6, Lower Yosemite Fall

Trail Use: Hiking, stroller accessible

Distance & Configuration: 2.0-mile loop

Elevation Range: 3,970 feet, with minimal elevation change

Facilities: You pass toilets, water taps, and picnic benches along the walk 0.1 mile beyond the shuttle stop. Snacks are available in Yosemite Lodge, 0.2 mile west along Yosemite Lodge Drive.

Highlights: Yosemite Valley views, meadows of tall grass, Merced River bridges, and a boardwalk

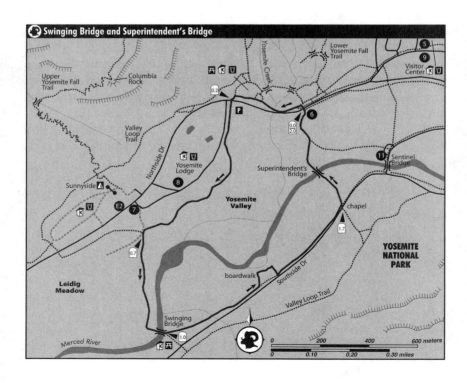

DESCRIPTION

This flat loop around Yosemite Valley is one of the best walks on which to absorb views of Half Dome and Yosemite Falls. Added bonuses are two beautiful bridges across the Merced River and a stretch of boardwalk through the valley's tall grass meadows. Mostly following a paved route, it is accessible to strollers.

THE ROUTE

From the shuttle stop, head west, crossing Yosemite Creek and passing the restrooms and picnic area until—across the street—you see the Yosemite Lodge parking area **(0.2 mile from start)**. Cross the street and walk along the sidewalk at the edge of Yosemite Lodge Drive for just 350 feet until you see a bike stand on your right. On the opposite side of the road, you will see two paved bike paths departing; the left-hand one is nearly perpendicular to the road, while the other diverges only slightly from the road. Take the right-hand choice.

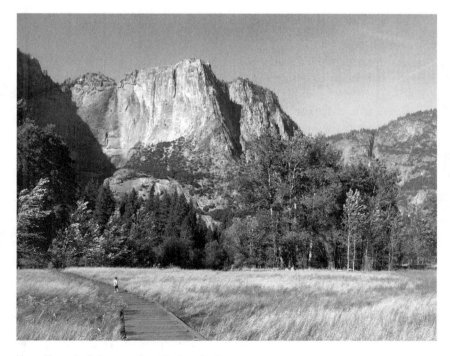

Upper Yosemite Fall as seen from the boardwalk

The bike path continues around the south side of Yosemite Lodge before trending left (south), where it approaches an out-of-service bus parking area **(0.7 mile)**. The trail now skirts the eastern edge of Leidig Meadow; this is a wonderful stretch of trail from which to stare to your southwest and admire the steep buttresses of Cathedral Rocks, while the Brothers dominate on the northern side of the valley. In spring this meadow is a vibrant green, while in autumn you gaze across a field of tall yellow stalks.

At the southern end of Leidig Meadow, you cross Swinging Bridge **(1.0 mile)**, a perfect location from which to gaze at Upper and Lower Yosemite falls—the Merced River and picturesque trees frame them. Beyond Swinging Bridge the trail turns east (left) and parallels Southside Drive (the valley road with eastbound traffic). The east end of the valley, and especially Half Dome, now dominate your view. Shortly, you pass a boardwalk that cuts into the meadow and then arcs back to meet the bike path a little farther ahead. I recommend this slight detour; it is delightful to walk through the otherwise off-limits meadow vegetation and to stare at the valley walls from the middle of a meadow.

Before long you see the Yosemite Chapel on the south side of the road and then reach a T-junction **(1.7 miles)**. Straight ahead the bike path continues to the east end of the valley, while the left-hand fork is a path that crosses Superintendent's Bridge and loops back to your shuttle stop—head left. Majestic black oaks shade much of the bridge, but their canopies don't quite meet in the middle, and shy squirrels race across the bridge once people are a *safe* distance away. A placard reminds you that the usually placid-looking river has severely flooded many times in the past century and will continue to do so. Once across the bridge, you follow the incense cedar–shaded path toward Northside Drive, ignoring a trail forking to the right and reaching the road in the vicinity of shuttle bus stop 6—cross the road to the shuttle stop **(2.0 miles)**.

TO THE TRAILHEAD

GPS Coordinates: N37° 44.744' W119° 35.623'

A limited amount of parking is available at Yosemite Lodge, but it is recommended that you take the Yosemite Valley Shuttle to the trailhead. Leave your car at your campsite or valley accommodation, or park at the large visitor parking lot at Yosemite Valley Shuttle stop 1. To reach this parking lot, drive east (toward Half Dome) on Southside Drive until you reach a stop sign at Sentinel Bridge, 4.1 miles from where CA 41 merges with Southside Drive. At this stop sign, straight ahead takes you to Curry

Village, while left across Sentinel Bridge leads to Yosemite Village and Yosemite Lodge. Turn left. After 0.3 mile, you reach a second stop sign; turning left takes you to Yosemite Lodge, while you turn right to Yosemite Village. Continue east for 0.1 mile to another stop sign and turn right into a large dirt parking area. Park your car and wait for the shuttle bus. Get off at stop 6, Lower Yosemite Fall.

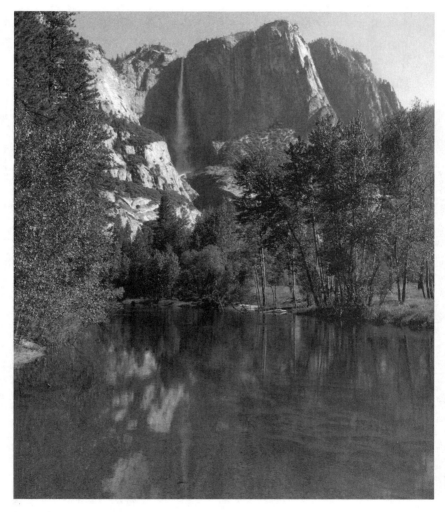

Upper Yosemite Fall viewed from Swinging Bridge

9   Mirror Lake

Trailhead Location: Yosemite Valley Shuttle stop 18, The Stables

Trail Use: Hiking

Distance & Configuration: 3.4-mile balloon

Elevation Range: 4,000 feet at the start, with a cumulative elevation change of ±200 feet

Facilities: You will pass water and toilets in the North Pines Campground as you begin your walk. Toilets are also at Mirror Lake.

Highlights: Vertical north face of Half Dome and Tenaya Canyon, as well as quiet forest and swimming holes

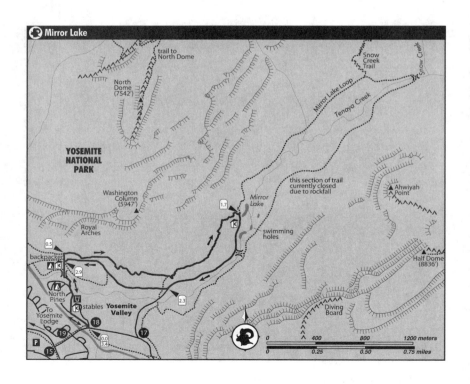

DESCRIPTION

This is a walk of contrasts—much of your walk is quiet, taking you along a less-used trail through tall conifer forests hugging the northern cliff faces at the east end of Yosemite Valley. When you reach Mirror Lake, the sense of enclosure is punctuated by expansive and stunning views of Tenaya Canyon and the north face of Half Dome—and a short time later your calm is interrupted by hordes of people marching up the paved Mirror Lake Trail to swim in one of two large water holes below the lake. Take this walk early in the day to avoid the crowds. This hike can be completed any time there isn't significant snow in Yosemite Valley.

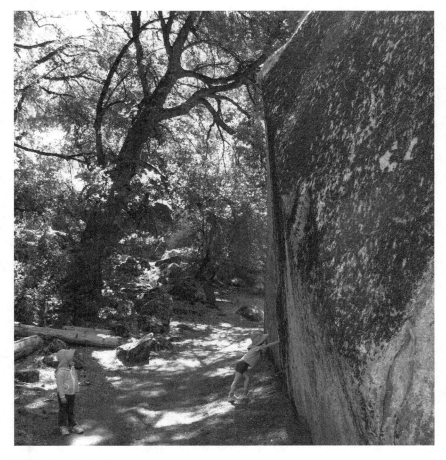

Enjoying the giant boulders

THE ROUTE

From the shuttle stop, turn right (north) onto the North Pines Campground entrance road, passing a kiosk and then entering the campground proper. Continue along the right-hand edge of the campground, following the one-way car route to the far back of the campground. Follow the trail that departs near site 331 and heads across Tenaya Creek to the backpacker campground. Continue through the backpacker campground to an X-junction with a paved bike path. Go straight ahead and immediately reach a T-junction with a dirt trail **(0.5 mile from start).** Turn right, toward Mirror Lake.

Other than the occasional pack train, this is a quiet trail. You are in a forest dominated by a handful of tall conifers, incense cedars, ponderosa pines, and a few sugar pines, as well as scattered live oaks and ubiquitous boulders. You sense the imposing valley walls not far to your left but see only glimpses of them as you pass first the Royal Arches and then the steep prow of Washington Column. A pile of giant moss-covered boulders, an old rockfall, is a reminder that Yosemite's vertical walls are forever shedding. Farther down the track are a few not too steep boulders that are a perfect playground for young children. Beyond, the trail bends slightly to the left and begins to climb gently. The forest is more open now, giving you more complete glimpses of Half Dome ahead and to your right and North Dome to your left. After passing through an open area, you descend briefly and reach a trail junction, where you turn right, cross a small bridge, and soon find yourself in front of Mirror Lake **(1.7 miles)**. The left fork takes you around the north side of Mirror Lake and an additional mile toward Tenaya Canyon. (The second half of the loop trail around Mirror Lake is indefinitely closed due to a rockslide of Ahwiyah Point, a sharp promontory to the northeast of Half Dome's face, so this trail is currently used mostly to access Snow Creek Trail.)

Within a few steps you see Mirror Lake ahead—or at least the dry expanse that is Mirror "Creek" in spring and early summer, for a lake only exists during floods. Head toward the shore and sit on boulders or beneath a tree for a quiet snack. The views up Tenaya Canyon are outstanding: to the left is the vertical face of Mount Watkins, to the right is the north face of Half Dome, and up canyon are the undulating polished granite slabs of Clouds Rest.

After absorbing the surroundings and having a snack, continue along the track and reach a spur up to a little alcove; it is currently decorated with all manner of rock towers—enjoy and contribute your own. Beyond you continue down to a restroom block, bicycle parking, and the first of the big swimming holes. In midsummer the relative sense of calm you enjoyed by the lake is quickly shattered by the happy screams of children playing in the water. Join in for a dip or continue down the now-paved trail, the main route to Mirror Lake. Remember that bicycles whiz down here, so stick to the side of the trail. Where the paved road begins to bend to the left, you will see a smaller bike path departing to the right—head right along it **(2.3 miles)**. You are now in the same forest as at the start of your walk, just 400 feet farther from the granite walls and on a large trail, giving you more of a sense of space. Remember to watch for bicycles as you walk back to the backpacker campground **(2.9 miles)** and then retrace your steps to the shuttle stop **(3.4 miles)**.

TO THE TRAILHEAD
GPS Coordinates: N37° 44.393' W119° 33.853'
The closest parking area is Curry Village (shuttle stops 14 and 20). To reach the parking lot, drive east (toward Half Dome) on Southside Drive. Along Southside Drive you will continue straight ahead at the first two stop signs you encounter: at a T-intersection at Sentinel Bridge, 4.1 miles east of where CA 41 from Wawona merges with the Valley loop, and at an X-intersection as you approach Curry Village, 1 mile east of Sentinel Bridge. After an additional 0.4 mile, turn right; you will immediately see a large parking area on your left. Pick a spot and head to shuttle bus stop 14, the bus stop on the east (parking lot side) of the road. Get off at stop 18, the Stables and North Pines campground stop—not stop 17, the Mirror Lake stop.

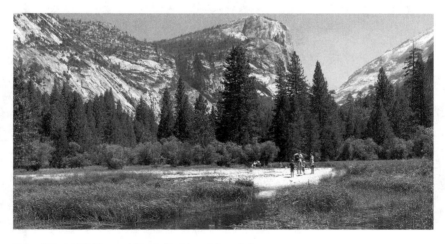

Vista of Mount Watkins and Clouds Rest from Mirror Lake

10 Base of Vernal Fall

Trailhead Location: Yosemite Valley Shuttle stop 16, Happy Isles

Trail Use: Hiking, stroller accessible with good breaks

Distance & Configuration: 2.2-mile out-and-back

Elevation Range: 4,020 feet at the start, with a cumulative elevation change of ±660 feet

Facilities: A drinking fountain and toilets are at shuttle stop 16 and also at the Vernal Fall Bridge, 0.9 mile into the walk. A snack bar is just behind the shuttle stop. If you have spare time before or after your walk, the Happy Isles Nature Center is excellent; children will especially enjoy the displays of Yosemite's animals. To reach it, head due south from the shuttle stop, instead of crossing the Merced River.

Highlights: Vernal Fall, walls below Glacier Point, and swirling waters of the Merced River

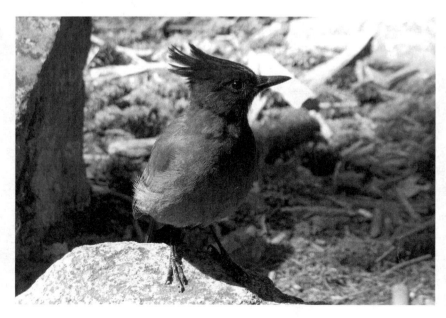

Steller's jay

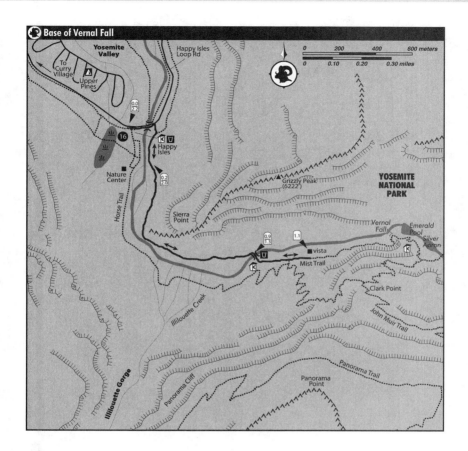

DESCRIPTION

If you can look past the crowds of people sharing the trail, you will discover yourself in a special corner of Yosemite Valley where the waterfalls and steep walls are in a very enclosed setting, making them feel even more all-encompassing and overpowering. The walking is easy but steep as you ascend the newly refurbished trail to the bridge below Vernal Fall. The waterfall is the highlight, but the walk is also impressive, for near-vertical walls surround you and the Merced River thunders beneath the trail.

THE ROUTE

Departing from the Happy Isles bus stop, you must first walk along the road's edge to cross the Merced River. The hiker's bridge across the river

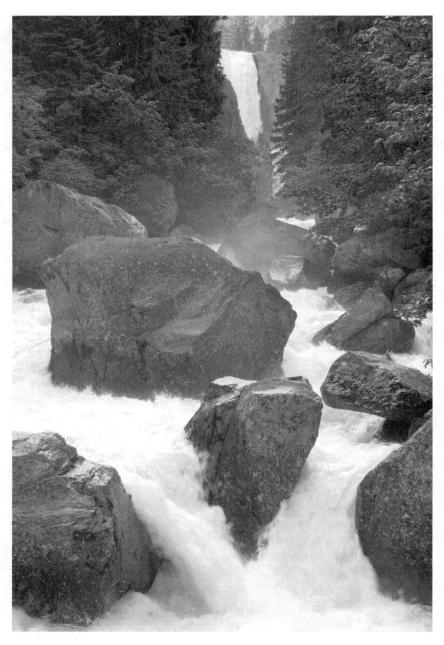

Vernal Fall

was washed out in floods in January 1997 and has not been replaced. Once across the river, turn right (south), descending to a broad dirt track that parallels the east riverbank. Shortly you pass a gauging station and the true trailhead **(0.2 mile from start)**, with a large sign indicating the distance to much farther destinations, for this is the start of the famous John Muir Trail and the hike up Half Dome.

The trail quickly enters forest cover—a mixture of conifers, deciduous trees, and, in patches, evergreen oaks—and begins to climb steadily. The trail's surface has been recently repaved, making it one of the few walks where pushing a stroller is feasible (and permitted as far as Vernal Fall Bridge), albeit a lot of work and a little scary on the descent.

Soon after passing a small spring enclosed by a lovely rock wall, you reach a corner with a must-see vista: far below, the Merced River is splashing over large rocks, while across the valley to the west is Glacier Point **(0.5 mile)**. Look at the light-colored rock near the top of the wall, a scar created during the large rockfall at Happy Isles in 1996. The steep scrubby walls to the east lead to pointy-topped Grizzly Peak and Sierra Point. Now trending east, the trail skirts around Sierra Point, with dramatic views down to the raging river (in spring) or giant polished boulders (in fall). To the south you look into Illilouette Gorge, with Illilouette Falls at its head. It is the least visited of Yosemite Valley's falls, for no trail accesses the amphitheater at its base.

Continuing up through a beautiful scrub oak forest and then across an open stretch of talus, debris left by an old rockfall, you descend briefly and see the bridge ahead **(0.9 mile)**. At most times you will be sharing the bridge with others, for everyone wants to watch the broad flow of Vernal Fall. In spring it spans the entire rock wall with a thick mass of water and spray, while in fall it is a thinner film of water. Both are attractive—early season for the overwhelming force and beauty of the waterfall and late season for the ability to see the beautifully polished and stained rocks that emerge from beneath the water.

If you wish to have a quieter spot to sit, there are several options. In fall you can climb down to the banks of the river and sit on boulders; they are most easily accessed from the north end of the bridge. If water levels are higher, continue up the trail a little. You will next come to a junction where the John Muir Trail is the right-hand choice and straight ahead is the Mist Trail. Continue up the Mist Trail just a short distance and you will see several places with large boulders on the river's bank; one particularly flat boulder has an outstanding view of Vernal Fall **(1.1 miles)**. To locate it, hunt for a chopped-off pole, and then note where a use trail descends through the rocks. Just be respectful of the water—it has enormous power and will quickly sweep you off your feet. Return to the shuttle stop by the same route **(2.2 miles)**.

TO THE TRAILHEAD

GPS Coordinates: N37° 43.949' W119° 33.559'

The closest parking area is Curry Village (shuttle stops 14 and 20). To reach the parking lot, drive east (toward Half Dome) on Southside Drive. Along Southside Drive you will continue straight ahead at the first two stop signs you encounter: at a T-intersection at Sentinel Bridge, 4.1 miles east of where CA 41 from Wawona merges with the Valley loop, and at an X-intersection as you approach Curry Village, 1 mile east of Sentinel Bridge. After an additional 0.4 mile, turn right; you will immediately see a large parking area on your left. Pick a spot and head to shuttle bus stop 14, the bus stop on the east (parking lot side) of the road. Get off at stop 16, Happy Isles.

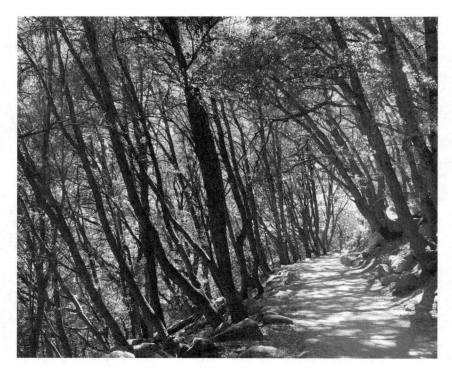

Trail through a scrub oak forest

11 Mist Trail and Clark Point

Trailhead Location: Yosemite Valley Shuttle stop 16, Happy Isles

Trail Use: Hiking

Distance & Configuration: 6.2-mile balloon (or 2.8-mile out-and-back to the top of Vernal Fall)

Elevation Range: 4,020 feet at the start, with a cumulative elevation change of ±2,150 feet

Facilities: A drinking fountain and toilets are at shuttle stop 16 and also at the Vernal Fall Bridge, 0.9 mile into the walk. A snack bar is just behind the shuttle stop. If you have spare time before or after your walk, the Happy Isles Nature Center is excellent; children will especially enjoy the displays of Yosemite's animals. To reach it, head due south from the shuttle stop instead of crossing the Merced River.

Highlights: Up, up, up alongside Vernal and Nevada falls; granite walls; and Half Dome views

DESCRIPTION

This justifiably popular loop climbs steeply beside Vernal and Nevada falls. The landscape is quite varied, including the drenching climb past Vernal Fall, dry flower-filled slopes, a well-walled traverse halfway up a granite cliff, and an aerial view of Vernal Fall. Note that the Mist Trail is closed in winter due to icy conditions.

THE ROUTE

Your route begins at the Happy Isles bus stop and continues first along the edge of the road, for the flood on January 2, 1997, washed out the footbridge upstream. After crossing the river, turn right and descend to a wide trail along the river's east bank. Beyond a marker indicating the height of the great flood, you reach a sign with mileages; you have reached the trailhead **(0.2 mile from start)**.

The broad paved path is well built to handle the considerable human traffic, for you are not the only one wishing to climb past two of Yosemite's iconic waterfalls. The route is steep but mostly well shaded as you encircle the out-of-sight summit of Grizzly Peak and Sierra Point, an old vista

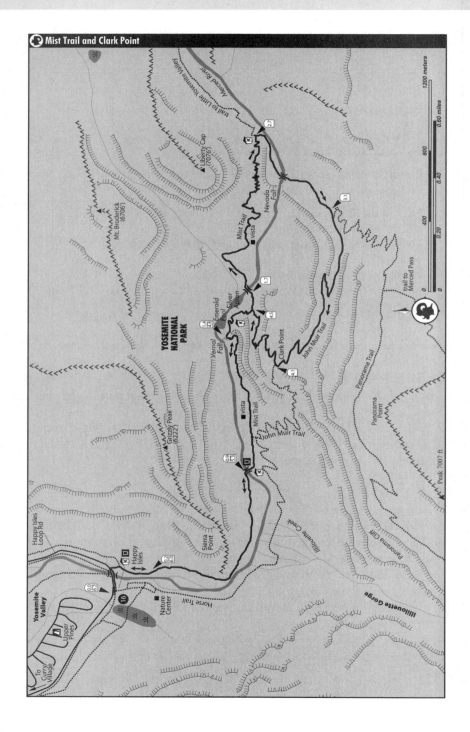

point halfway up the peak. Where you reach a sharp turn to the left, stop and look over the edge of the tall rock wall. Below the Merced River is tumbling over large boulders, and to your west are the steep granite walls leading up to Glacier Point. To the south is the amphitheater holding Illilouette Falls. Continuing up, first beneath a beautiful grove of scrub oak and then an open talus slope, you descend briefly and immediately turn right to cross the Merced River **(0.9 mile)**. Here you will undoubtedly join everyone else and photograph Vernal Fall. In spring the waterfall covers the entire rock wall with a thick mass of water and spray, while in fall a thinner line of water descends, allowing you to see the stained and polished rock behind.

Passing a water fountain and restrooms, the trail turns left and resumes its ascent beneath tall Douglas firs to a junction where you continue straight ahead, up the Mist Trail to the top of Vernal Fall and then Nevada Fall; the right-hand fork is the John Muir Trail and an alternative route up. You continue along the riverbank, leaving forest cover and following the trail across steep granite slabs. Ahead, the grade steepens into a staircase and the grass on the slope becomes a very vibrant green due to continuous spray from the falls; *vernal* is the perfect description. In spring many people choose to wear a poncho on this ascent, for you will reach the top wet, but I find that I heat up quite enough on the climb and don't mind the moisture.

The stairs continue relentlessly and even increase in height toward the top. Just keep stopping to take photographs, for the view of the waterfall is simply superb. Finally the stairs end and the trail traverses left on a narrow (and fenced) ledge, bringing you to the top of the fall **(1.4 miles)**. After the requisite peer over the safety railing and a break, follow the bank of the river upstream—the trail becomes obvious again where you leave the slabs. Pass the beautifully colored Emerald Pool on your left and a toilet to the right, and then turn and climb up a few switchbacks to a junction. Stay left (you will come down the right-hand fork later), traverse an open slab, and then cross the Silver Apron Bridge **(1.7 miles)**. This bridge also needed to be rebuilt after the 1997 flood.

A brief ascent takes you to a flat shelf, at the end of which the trail bends left. Before marching onward, detour briefly to the south (toward the river), for this is a spectacular location from which to view Nevada Fall. Then retreat to the trail, switchback upward first under forest cover to the base of Liberty Cap, and then up a steep, dry, open slope beneath vertical granite walls. In spring abundant wildflowers will likely keep you entertained, but this section is a tough climb—your legs are already tired and

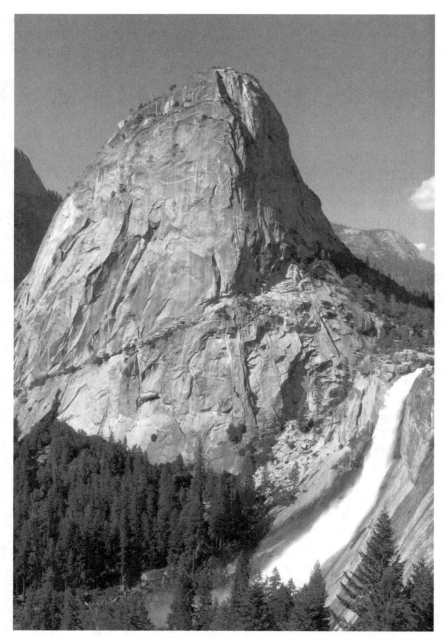

Liberty Cap and Nevada Fall

the grade is relentless. Finally two tight switchbacks alongside a tall wall bring you to a junction beside a toilet **(2.7 miles)**.

Instead of taking your break here, turn right onto the John Muir Trail toward Yosemite Valley and climb briefly to the true top of Nevada Fall. You emerge beside the Merced River on an open slab lined with boulders and then reach a bridge. Before crossing the bridge, head right to a fenced lookout and enjoy a snack on the river's bank. And be smart—stay behind the fence and don't swim in the river upstream of the waterfall, for people really do fall to their deaths.

Climbing briefly through a forest, you reach, in quick succession, two junctions with the Panorama Trail **(3.1 miles)**. Stay right each time and you will soon find yourself on a walled-in ledge high on the cliff face to the south of Nevada Fall. The view to the fall and to the domes behind is spectacular. Half Dome is in the background with Mount Broderick and Liberty Cap in front. Continue switchbacking down, entering open forest with each westward length and enjoying views of Nevada Fall during east-ward trajectories, until you reach the Clark Point vista and another junction **(4.1 miles)**. The John Muir Trail continues down the left-hand fork, while you should take the right-hand fork down a less-used trail that loops back to the top of Vernal Fall.

This short connector trail descends directly above Vernal Fall, with one particularly good near-aerial view of the falls—be aware that no safety fence exists here, so watch your footing. Below you reach the trail junction above Vernal Fall that you passed earlier **(4.5 miles)**. Turn left and retrace your steps from here to the shuttle bus stop **(6.2 miles)**.

TO THE TRAILHEAD
GPS Coordinates: N37° 43.949' W119° 33.559'
The closest parking area is Curry Village (shuttle stops 14 and 20). To reach the parking lot, drive east (toward Half Dome) on Southside Drive. Along Southside Drive you will continue straight ahead at the first two stop signs you encounter: at a T-intersection at Sentinel Bridge, 4.1 miles east of where CA 41 from Wawona merges with the Valley loop, and at an X-intersection as you approach Curry Village, 1 mile east of Sentinel Bridge. After an additional 0.4 mile, turn right; you will immediately see a large parking area on your left. Pick a spot and head to shuttle bus stop 14, the bus stop on the east side (parking lot side) of the road. Get off at stop 16, Happy Isles.

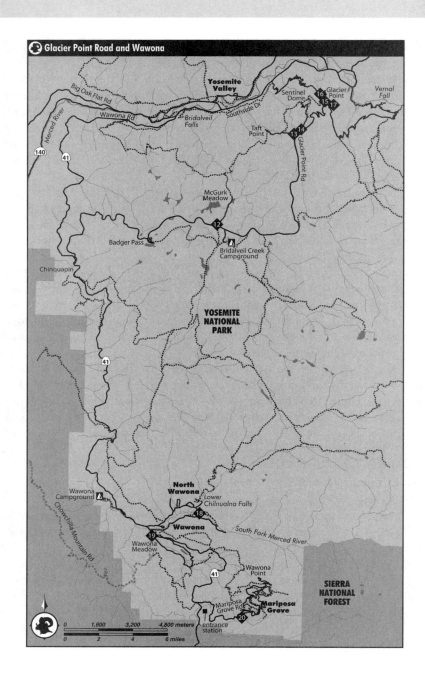

GLACIER POINT ROAD AND WAWONA

Regional Overview

This section includes hikes from southwestern Yosemite, a more forested region with fewer of the striking summits and vistas that define most of the park. But treasures abound, including striking wildflower displays, beautiful conifer forests, the largest of Yosemite's giant sequoia groves, cascading waterfalls, and of course lots of granite slabs, domes, and cliffs. To the north, the southern rim of Yosemite Valley, with its striking view of the incomparable valley, bounds this region.

The hikes included provide a sampling of all the area's highlights, with a bit of a bias to valley rim views, for each lookout is situated differently and all are worth enjoying. The abundant water and relatively flat topography in the vicinity of Glacier Point Road make this a prime location for colorful summer wildflower displays (and mosquitoes). Here I have included only McGurk Meadow (Hike 12), generally considered the most spectacular and one that is easy to reach. If you are awed by the flowers, consider Westfall Meadows, Mono Meadows, and Lost Bear Meadow as future destinations. Wawona Meadow (Hike 19) is another favorite wildflower hike and one showcasing both spring and summer wildflowers at a lower elevation.

Of the walks described here, Sentinel Dome (Hike 14) and Glacier Point (Hike 15) are the most recommended family destinations. On my last ascent of Sentinel Dome, our family was one of four on the summit with children under age 5; the kids had all raced up the slabs and were scrambling on the boulders near the summit. Taft Point (Hike 13) is also within a 5-year-old's range, but the lack of a safe viewing platform would make me uneasy. The lower reaches of Mariposa Grove (Hike 20) are a good choice for young children, while an 8-year-old could complete the

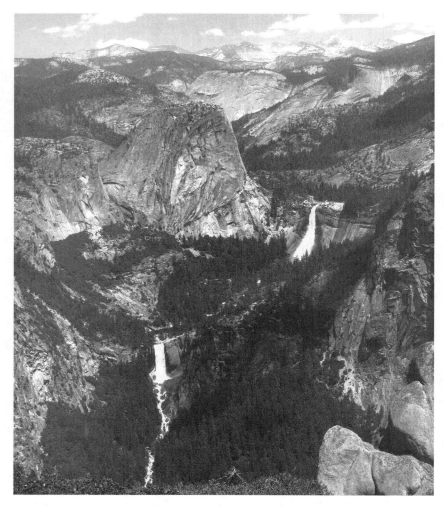

Vernal and Nevada falls from the Panorama Trail (see page 91)

entire loop described. Do note that this is a particularly hot location mid-summer. If you are reasonably sure that the mosquito season is past its worst, McGurk Meadow (Hike 12) and Wawona Meadow (Hike 19) also make good family destinations for finding a rainbow of flowers.

◘   ◘   ◘

12 McGurk Meadow

Trailhead Location: Glacier Point Road, near Bridalveil Creek Campground

Trail Use: Hiking

Distance & Configuration: 2.0-mile out-and-back

Elevation Range: 7,040 feet at the start, with a cumulative elevation change of ±280 feet

Facilities: No amenities are at the trailhead, but toilets and water are available in Bridalveil Creek Campground.

Highlights: Colorful expanses of wildflowers, large marshy meadow, and a quiet forest walk

DESCRIPTION

McGurk Meadow is justifiably well known for its exquisite wildflower displays; there are both many species and such an abundance of some species that they create brilliant patches of color. A flat, shaded walk leads to the meadow, which is dissected by a picturesque meandering creek. In early summer the mosquitoes may be as abundant as the wildflowers, so bring insect repellent.

THE ROUTE

Leaving Glacier Point Road, you immediately enter a dense fir pine forest with lush understory, remarkably green through much of the summer. The nearly flat trail makes for fast walking as you enjoy the abundant wildflowers and step across a seasonal trickle. Notice all the dead branches on the trees; this patch of forest has not been burnt for many years, allowing the build-up of dead wood.

Shortly, you reach an imperceptible saddle and descend to McGurk Meadow. You pass an old cabin, built in the 1890s by herder John McGurk, and just beyond you enter the meadow **(0.7 mile from start)**. The stream, a tributary of Bridalveil Creek, meanders through the marshy meadow, and long after spring has left most of Yosemite, McGurk Meadow still glows a particularly vibrant light green. Ahead, a bridge crosses the main creek channel. Beyond, rocks line the edge,

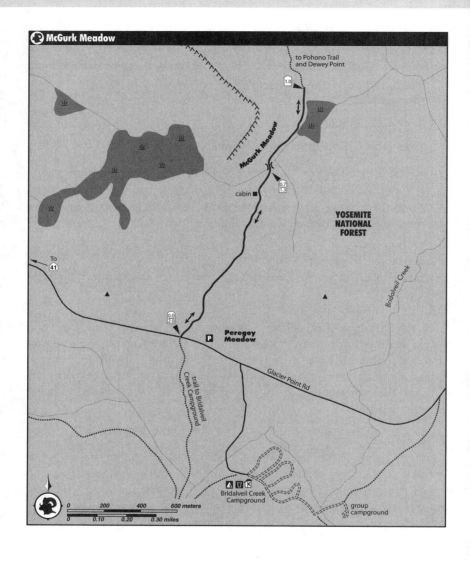

allowing you to stay out of the often-muddy trail. Stop on the bridge and enjoy your mid-meadow view that extends up and down a long narrow stretch of McGurk Meadow; farther upstream (to your left, west) the meadow becomes broader and even marshier.

From the bridge you will likely notice the bright patches of flowers dotting the meadow. Right along the stream bank are rows of white western bistorts. Just beyond are expanses of lilac shooting stars. Even drier stretches of meadow may be orange with paintbrushes or dark purple with lupines. To enjoy these and many of the other species that grow in the meadow, continue along the trail until you leave the meadow **(1.0 mile)**, for you will pass many different species. As you walk across and then along the meadow, there are continuous changes in soil moisture and temperature, indiscernible to us, but each plant has its own preferred habitat and many species appear in just one spot along the trail. As you explore, stick to the trail, for walking on the meadow, especially when soggy, compacts the soil and tramples the plants. Return the way you came **(2.0 miles)**.

TO THE TRAILHEAD
GPS Coordinates: N37° 40.226' W119° 37.692'
From Yosemite Valley, head to the location where Southside Drive, the eastbound road in Yosemite Valley, and CA 41, the road from Wawona, meet. If you are in Yosemite Village or Curry Village, this requires taking westbound Northside Drive to the western end of the valley. Stay in the left lane to cross the Merced River. After 0.9 mile you will reach the CA

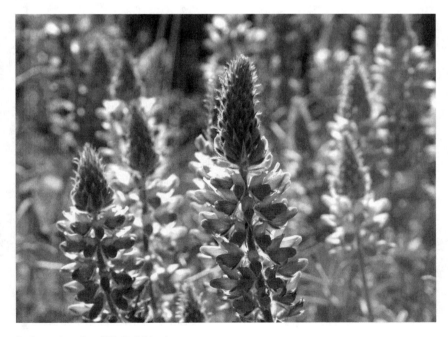

Lupine at the edge of McGurk Meadow

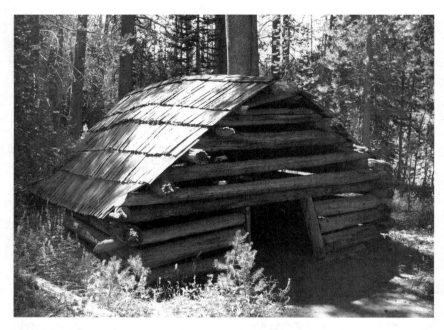

John McGurk's cabin

41 junction and turn right onto CA 41. Continue for 9.2 miles, passing through the Wawona Tunnel and eventually reaching a left-hand junction. Straight ahead takes you to Wawona, while you turn left onto Glacier Point Road. Continue 7.7 miles to a small parking area on the left (north) side of the road, a little west of the entrance road to Bridalveil Creek Campground. After you park, head west along the road for 500 feet to the start of the trail. (The turnoff to Glacier Point Road is 12.3 miles north of Wawona.)

13 Taft Point

Trailhead Location: Glacier Point Road, 1.9 miles before Glacier Point

Trail Use: Hiking

Distance & Configuration: 2.4-mile out-and-back

Elevation Range: 7,720 feet at the start, with a cumulative elevation change of ±440 feet

Facilities: Toilets are at the trailhead. Water is available at Glacier Point and in the Bridalveil Creek Campground.

Highlights: The Fissures, overhanging vista of El Capitan, and wildflowers

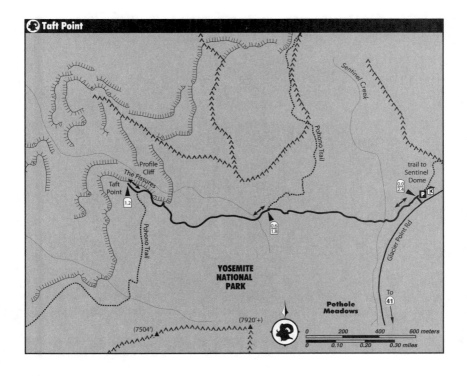

DESCRIPTION

This short walk combines many attractions, most notably the panoramic vista of western Yosemite Valley from Taft Point and the several deep clefts in the granite rim known as the Fissures. En route the trail borders flower-filled creek banks, an unexpected bonus for most hikers. In distance and elevation gain the walk is appropriate for children, but neither the Fissures nor Taft Point offer a barrier, making this a potentially dangerous destination.

THE ROUTE

Descending a spur trail just right of the toilets, you quickly reach a T-junction with the main trail and turn left (south). Initially paralleling the road, you pass an impressively large outcrop of bright white quartz and then turn right (west) and descend to Sentinel Creek. During low water it is an easy step across; otherwise you can balance across some small logs bridging the channel. Climbing now, you enter an open, sandy flat dotted with white mariposa lilies in early summer. *Mariposa* is Spanish for "butterfly," and these flowers are named for their white petals, shaped like butterfly

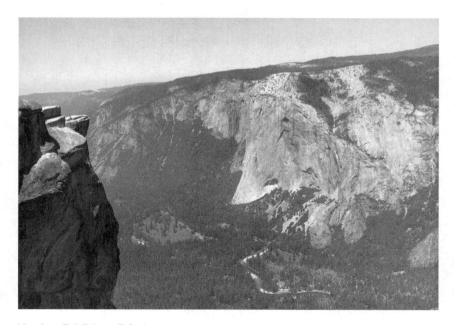

View from Taft Point to El Capitan

wings and decorated with colorful markings. Dropping just slightly you enter a patch of denser forest and then climb again into open landscape. Large trees, especially some impressively large Jeffrey pines, dot the landscape. Descending again you reach a trail junction, where you take the left branch to Taft Point, while the right branch is the Pohono Trail that leads to Sentinel Dome and Glacier Point **(0.6 mile from start)**.

You now begin a steady descent to the rim of Yosemite Valley, first passing through lovely patches of wildflowers lining the banks of an unnamed trickle. Light purple shooting stars, darker purple lupines, yellow groundsels, orange alpine lilies, and tall white corn lilies are all present, creating dense bursts of color in the early and midsummer. After climbing in and out of several of these lush wildflower gardens, the forest opens and you are at the top of a slope of granite slabs broken by patches of shallow sandy soil. The trail descends the right-hand edge of the slope; walk slowly, for the sand-covered rock is slippery.

Where the slope lessens, the track continues straight ahead, but you repeatedly notice footprints heading off to the right, where a steep narrow gorge has swallowed the little creek you crossed higher up. The entrance to the ravine, located just 100 feet to the right of the trail, marks the start of Profile Cliff, a vertical face interrupted by five long, narrow chasms, known as the Fissures. These cracks exist along joint lines, widespread fractures that extend across vast distances in Yosemite and are responsible for many nearby vertical landscape features, including Yosemite Valley itself and the face of Half Dome. The most impressive of the Fissures are just before your final ascent to the Taft Point lookout—here the cracks are the longest, and two wedged boulders can be found in one. As you peer into the abysses, remember that sand-covered granite is slippery and step carefully.

When you are finished staring down, look back up and note an old barrier indicating the lookout a short distance above you. The Pohono Trail now bends left, continuing west along the valley rim, and you leave the trail to go right and climb up slabs to the overhanging overlook **(1.2 miles)**. The views in all directions are impressive, although I am most awed by looking straight across at the 3,000-foot vertical face of El Capitan. The view right (eastward) extends to Yosemite Falls. (Note that Taft Point itself lies 0.1 mile northwest of the railing, but most people choose to admire the valley from this slightly protected location.)

When you are finished, return the way you came **(2.4 miles)**. For a longer option not described in this book, you can continue east along the Pohono Trail and eventually up Sentinel Dome. From Sentinel Dome return to your car as described in Hike 14 **(total distance 5.4 miles)**.

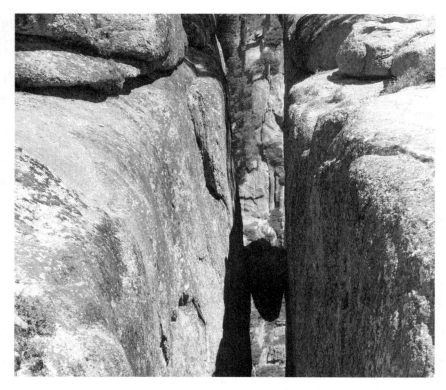

One of the Fissures

TO THE TRAILHEAD

GPS Coordinates: N37° 42.741' W119° 35.190'

From Yosemite Valley, head to the location where Southside Drive, the eastbound road in the valley, and CA 41, the road from Wawona, meet. If you are in Yosemite Village or Curry Village, this requires taking westbound Northside Drive to the western end of the valley. Stay in the left lane to cross the Merced River. After 0.9 mile you will reach the CA 41 junction and turn right onto CA 41. Continue for 9.2 miles, passing through the Wawona Tunnel and eventually reaching a left-hand junction. Straight ahead takes you to Wawona, while you turn left onto Glacier Point Road. Continue 13.4 miles to a small parking area on the left (west) side of the road; this is also the parking area for the hike to Sentinel Dome. Alternatively drive 1.9 miles west from Glacier Point. (The turnoff to Glacier Point Road is 12.3 miles north of Wawona.)

14 Sentinel Dome

Trailhead Location: Glacier Point Road, 1.9 miles before Glacier Point

Trail Use: Hiking

Distance & Configuration: 2.2-mile out-and-back

Elevation Range: 7,720 feet at the start to 8,122 feet at the summit, with a cumulative elevation change of ±580 feet

Facilities: Toilets are at the trailhead. Water is available at Glacier Point and in the Bridalveil Creek Campground.

Highlights: Granite slab summit, stunted trees, and expansive Yosemite high-country vista

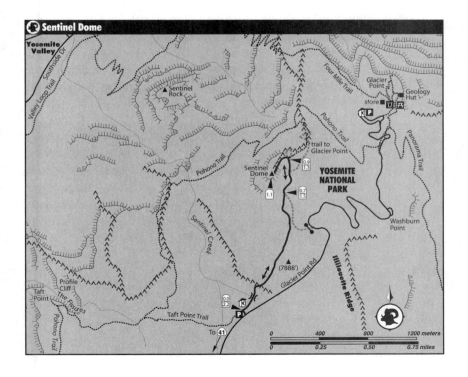

DESCRIPTION

The hike to Sentinel Dome is one of Yosemite's easiest summit hikes, making it a fantastic destination for children. A beautiful summit, it is sufficiently higher than Glacier Point, so the view includes more of the high peaks in the eastern part of Yosemite and is simply an enjoyable spot to take an extended break.

THE ROUTE

Descend behind the restrooms to the main trail and then head right (north). The landscape is quite open, with intermittent views to the west broken by stands of trees. At first the trail parallels Glacier Point Road, but fortunately the trail is sufficiently down an escarpment to dull the traffic noise. Soon it diverges from the road, crosses a small creek on a wooden bridge, and skirts around the western side of a small dome. You now begin a gradual ascent up sandy slabs surrounded by low-growing bushes, huckleberry oaks, and pinemat manzanitas, with a view to Sentinel Dome just ahead. Beyond, you reach a trail junction **(0.7 mile from start)**, where straight ahead leads to Sentinel Dome, and the right-hand branch, a closed service road, leads back to Glacier Point Road at a secondary (and unmarked) parking area.

Skirting the east side of Sentinel Dome, you are walking through an open forest of mature conifers—red firs with their rich red bark; the fine, flaky bark of lodgepole pines; and scattered Jeffrey pines with notably

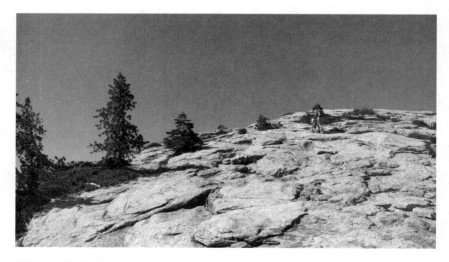

Walking up Sentinel Dome

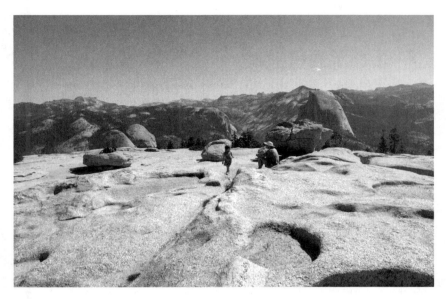

From the summit, view to Half Dome and Tenaya Canyon

long branches and needles. You next reach a junction where you continue straight ahead, and almost immediately you reach a second junction, where right (northeast) leads down to Glacier Point, Washburn Point, and the Pohono Trail to Taft Point, and left (southwest) leads up Sentinel Dome **(0.9 mile)**.

You quickly emerge from forest cover and begin to ascend a sandy slope that transitions to slabs. There is no longer a distinct trail, but abundant footprints in the sand and cairns (rock piles) mark the way to the summit. Take care on the sand- and gravel-covered slabs, as your feet can easily slip from under you—nice circular sand grains on smooth rock can be nearly as dangerous as marbles on a floor. Glaciers did not polish the rock atop Sentinel Dome; it instead formed by exfoliation, or the flaking off of concentric layers of rock, a process that creates many of Yosemite's lower elevation domes.

As you ascend, you can enjoy the ever-expanding panorama. Yosemite Falls is now visible across Yosemite Valley, and the tall peaks in eastern Yosemite are prominent on the horizon. Before long, you find yourself on the summit, often a blustery location **(1.1 miles)**. Locate a large boulder on which is mounted a placard identifying many of

Yosemite's summits. Take the time to identify Mount Lyell, Yosemite's high point, and Mount Hoffmann, the geographical center of the park (and Hike 26). Looking west provides a view of Yosemite Valley and, on a clear day, all the way to the Coast Ranges. Wander around and admire the stunted Jeffrey pines that survive on the summit, their roots stuck in cracks holding the only available soil.

After a lengthy break, retrace your steps to the car **(2.2 miles)**. Note that this hike can be combined with Hike 13, Taft Point, into a 5.4-mile loop by heading downslope at the junction 0.2 mile before the summit. The route is shown on the map for this hike.

TO THE TRAILHEAD
GPS Coordinates: N37° 42.741' W119° 35.190'
Head to the location in Yosemite Valley where Southside Drive, the eastbound road in the valley, and CA 41, the road from Wawona, meet. If you are in Yosemite Village or Curry Village, this requires taking westbound Northside Drive to the western end of the valley. Stay in the left lane to cross the Merced River. After 0.9 mile you will reach the CA 41 junction and turn right onto CA 41. Continue for 9.2 miles, passing through the Wawona Tunnel and eventually reaching a left-hand junction. Straight ahead takes you to Wawona, while you turn left onto Glacier Point Road. Continue 13.4 miles to a small parking area on the left (west) side of the road; this is also the parking area for the hike to Taft Point. Alternatively drive 1.9 miles west from Glacier Point. (The turnoff to Glacier Point Road is 12.3 miles north of Wawona.)

15 Glacier Point

Trailhead Location: Glacier Point parking lot

Trail Use: Hiking, stroller accessible

Distance & Configuration: 0.6-mile balloon

Elevation Range: 7,190 feet at the start, with a cumulative elevation change of ±25 feet

Facilities: Amenities include a snack bar, toilets (parking area only), and water (parking area and snack bar).

Highlights: Aerial views of Yosemite Valley and beyond, granite in all directions, and glacial history

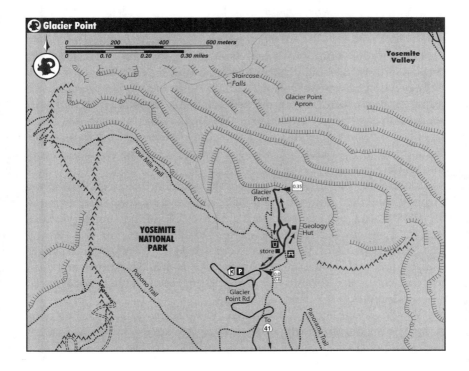

DESCRIPTION

The vista point is simply phenomenal. You can look straight down on the eastern half of Yosemite Valley (and Yosemite Falls) or east to Half Dome and the amphitheater containing Nevada and Vernal falls. The attraction is the enormity of the view, not just gushing waterfalls in spring, making this a must-visit location any time Glacier Point Road is open, usually mid-May–October. During the middle of the day in summer, Glacier Point is very crowded. It is advisable to visit early in the morning, when you can sit quietly and absorb the enormity of the landscape, or at sunset, the time of day with the best lighting. Once you have driven all the way to Glacier Point, you may want to include a second nearby trail in your itinerary. McGurk Meadow (Hike 12), Sentinel Dome (Hike 14), and Taft Point (Hike 13) are all excellent choices.

THE ROUTE

From the parking area, pass the toilets and continue along a paved trail to a wide patio. The snack bar is on your left, and an amphitheater on your right is a lovely and usually not too crowded place to sit. Bend left to continue to Glacier Point. After 100 feet you reach an X-junction, where the right-hand fork takes you to the Geology Hut, straight ahead leads directly to Glacier Point, and the left-hand fork is an alternative, wheelchair- and stroller-accessible route to Glacier Point (and Four Mile Trail, Hike 16, branches off it). Bear right to the Geology Hut, an excellent display partially enclosed by rock walls. Look at the sketches of a glacier-covered landscape and then turn around and stare at the mountains, imagining the nearby domes buried under ice while the higher sharper-summited peaks remained snow free. The Geology Hut is also a good location to admire the eastward view: Half Dome, Vernal and Nevada falls, and the tall peaks of southeastern Yosemite beyond.

Continuing north, you loop back to the main paved trail, where you turn right and then continue straight ahead (north) until you see the ground disappear ahead—you have reached the rim **(0.35 mile from start)**. Rock walls and railings line the edge, so there is ample space for safe viewing from this overhanging vista point. Yosemite Falls, North Dome, Tenaya Canyon, and Half Dome are laid out in front of you. Be sensible, and don't try to reach some of the outlying pinnacles, instead enjoying the photos of pioneers in petticoats balancing on them.

When you are done absorbing the view, return to the parking area, taking the main trail straight south to the snack bar and then bearing right (west), retracing your steps **(0.6 mile)**.

TO THE TRAILHEAD

GPS Coordinates: N37° 43.661' W119° 34.462'

From Yosemite Valley, head to the location where Southside Drive, the eastbound road in the valley, and CA 41, the road from Wawona, meet. If you are in Yosemite Village or Curry Village, this requires taking westbound Northside Drive to the western end of the valley. Stay in the left lane to cross the Merced River. After 0.9 mile you will reach the CA 41 junction and turn right onto CA 41. Continue for 9.2 miles, passing through the Wawona Tunnel and eventually reaching a left-hand junction. Straight ahead takes you to Wawona, while you turn left onto Glacier Point Road. Continue 15.3 miles to the end of the road and the Glacier Point parking lot. (The turnoff to Glacier Point Road is 12.3 miles north of Wawona.) If you do not want to drive, a commercial bus departs from Yosemite Lodge three times daily for a 4-hour tour to Glacier Point. See **yosemitepark.com** for more information on Glacier Point tours.

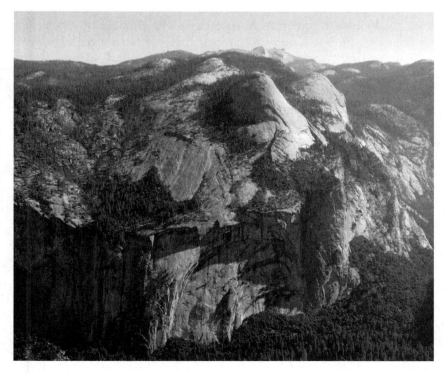

Scenic view to Royal Arches and North Dome

16 Four Mile Trail

Trailhead Location: Glacier Point parking lot

Trail Use: Hiking

Distance & Configuration: 4.8-mile point to point

Elevation Range: 7,190 feet at the start to 3,980 at the end, with a cumulative descent of 3,300 feet

Facilities: A snack bar, toilets (parking area only), and water (parking area and snack bar) are at Glacier Point.

Highlights: Long downhill and extensive and varied Yosemite Valley views, especially Yosemite Falls

DESCRIPTION

Yosemite Valley's features change appearance with elevation above the valley floor and are best absorbed by viewing them from above, below, and straight on. Unless you are a rock climber, the Four Mile Trail provides the best location to complete this task. It follows a path of nearly continuous views from Glacier Point, on the south rim, to Yosemite Valley and lies directly across from Yosemite Falls. Thanks to a convenient, albeit pricey, tour bus from Yosemite Valley to Glacier Point, this one-way hike can be completed without any logistical difficulty.

THE ROUTE

Once off the bus at the Glacier Point parking area, head north along the wide paved trail toward the snack hut. Just beyond you reach a junction, where straight ahead leads to Glacier Point (Hike 15), but you turn left and descend a length of stairs. (If you have never been to Glacier Point, budget 15 minutes and an additional 0.4 mile to walk to the rim and peer over, for the views toward Half Dome are not as satisfying from the Four Mile Trail, where Vernal and Nevada falls are hidden.) You descend a short distance before leveling out beneath dense forest cover, stepping across a small stream, and continuing on a northwesterly trajectory.

A steep cliff face lies not far to your right (northeast), but trees mostly block the landscape until you emerge onto a rock ledge **(0.5 mile from start)**. Suddenly you have wonderful views across Yosemite Valley to Royal

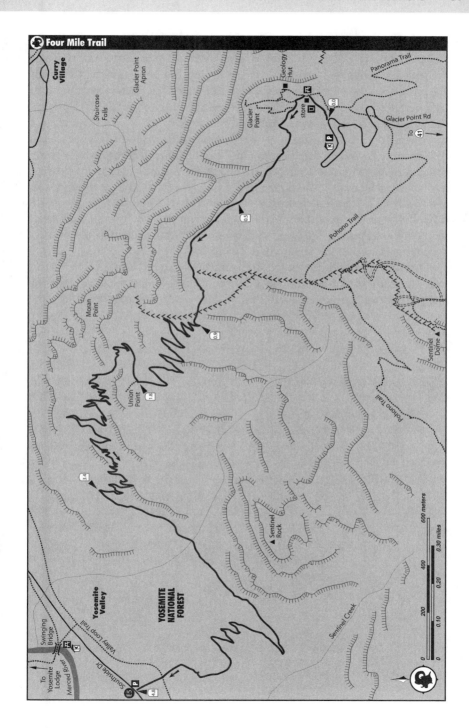

Four Mile Trail

Arches, North Dome, and Yosemite Falls and can also see up Tenaya Canyon to the east. This is a hike of evolving views—you may think that you are walking straight down to Yosemite Valley, but there is actually a considerable amount of westward sidling. For this first stretch of trail, your views are to the northeast, while later, once you have rounded Moran Point, the western half of Yosemite Valley dominates.

Soon you are again heading west among shrubs and under scattered tree cover, and once past the unseen Moran Point **(0.9 mile)**, you begin the endlessly switchbacking descent. First are a series of zigzags down a dry slope with tall shrubs and limited views. The ground here is quite soft, as soil actually overlays the rocks. The switchbacks end at a junction **(1.8 miles)**, where the main trail turns to the right and a left-hand fork takes you to Union Point. It is a beautiful viewpoint, but not much different from panoramas you will see lower down the trail, so bear right.

The trail now bends east (right) to traverse a steep forested slope into a passable gully between Union and Moran points. Enjoy the shade, for the rest of the trail is more exposed and hotter. Where topography allows, the

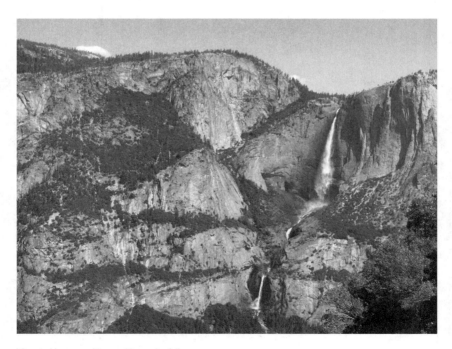

View to Upper and Lower Yosemite falls

trail sneaks west again, skirting around the ridge that descends from Union Point. Rounding the corner, you begin 1,200 feet of switchbacks straight down a scrubby slope.

The trail here is rocky—walk slowly, for the gravel on underlying rocks is slippery and the nonstop pounding is difficult on your feet. Oak trees provide occasional shade but mostly just obscure your never-ending and absolutely phenomenal view to Yosemite Falls. The best landscape views tend to be at the mid-elevations, where you are looking across, not up or down, and right here you are staring straight at the middle of Yosemite Falls and many of Yosemite's enormous walls of granite. Equally breath-taking are the views to the western end of Yosemite Valley: the Cathedral Rocks on the left and El Capitan on the right, separated by the flat expanse of tall trees on the valley floor.

The trail's grade doesn't decrease, but eventually the switchbacks end and you begin a long westward traverse to a more gradual slope **(3.4 miles)**. You continue enjoying the views until you reenter a mixed conifer and oak forest and descend a final series of switchbacks to the valley floor **(4.8 miles)**.

TO THE TRAILHEAD

GPS Coordinates:
Glacier Point parking lot: N37° 43.661' W119° 34.462'
Four Mile Trailhead: N37° 43.949' W119° 33.559'
If you plan to do a car shuttle or have someone drop you at Glacier Point, see Glacier Point (Hike 15) for driving directions. A few parking spots are at the trail's end, the Four Mile Trailhead in Yosemite Valley, to leave a car to retrieve on your return. A logistically easier alternative is to take a tour bus from Yosemite Lodge to Glacier Point. Park your car at your Yosemite Valley accommodation or at the large Yosemite Village visitor parking lot (shuttle stop 1) and take the Valley shuttle to Yosemite Lodge (stop 8). If you are driving from outside the valley, to reach the parking lot, drive east (toward Half Dome) on Southside Drive, until you reach Sentinel Bridge, 4.1 miles from where CA 41 merges with Valley Loop Road and your first stop sign. Straight ahead takes you to Curry Village, while turning left takes you across Sentinel Bridge to Yosemite Village and Yosemite Lodge. After 0.3 mile you reach a second stop sign; turning left takes you to Yosemite Lodge, while you turn right to Yosemite Village. Continue east for 0.1 mile to another stop sign and turn right into a large dirt parking area.

At the end of the day, you will again use shuttles to return to your car. Mid-June–early September the free El Capitan shuttle bus stops at the

Four Mile Trailhead until 6 p.m., looping back to the Valley Visitor Center (El Capitan shuttle stop 1) or Yosemite Lodge (El Capitan shuttle stop 2), where you can transfer to the Valley shuttle. Then use the Valley shuttle to reach your car, campsite, or lodging. During other months you must either have shuttled a car to the Four Mile Trailhead or you must walk 0.9 mile back to Yosemite Lodge. To do this, first turn right (east) and follow the Valley Loop Trail to Swinging Bridge. Cross Swinging Bridge and follow the paved bike path to Yosemite Lodge, where the Valley shuttle stops year-round. (See **nps.gov/yose/planyourvisit/bus.htm** for additional information on all buses described.)

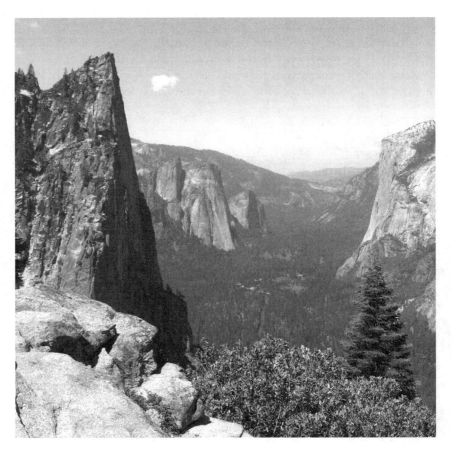

Looking west to the Cathedral Rocks and El Capitan

17 Panorama Trail

Trailhead Location: Glacier Point parking lot

Trail Use: Hiking

Distance & Configuration: 8.2-mile point to point

Elevation Range: 7,190 feet at the start to 4,020 at the end, with a cumulative ascent of 640 feet and descent of 4,430 feet

Facilities: A snack bar, toilets (parking area only), and water (parking area and snack bar) are at Glacier Point.

Highlights: Waterfalls, vistas, more waterfalls, more vistas

DESCRIPTION

The Panorama Trail's name provides the necessary description: this is Yosemite Valley's most view-rich walk. The trail descends from Glacier Point to Yosemite Valley via Illilouette, Nevada, and Vernal falls, providing nearly continuous vistas into and across the Merced River Canyon and the east end of Yosemite Valley. It is especially rewarding, for as it traverses eastward, it provides ever-changing views of the surrounding walls, waterfalls, and canyon.

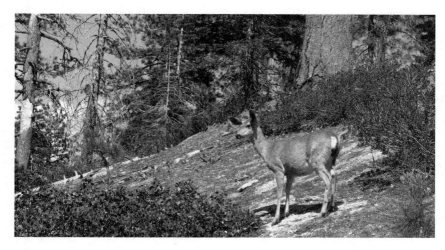

A mule deer

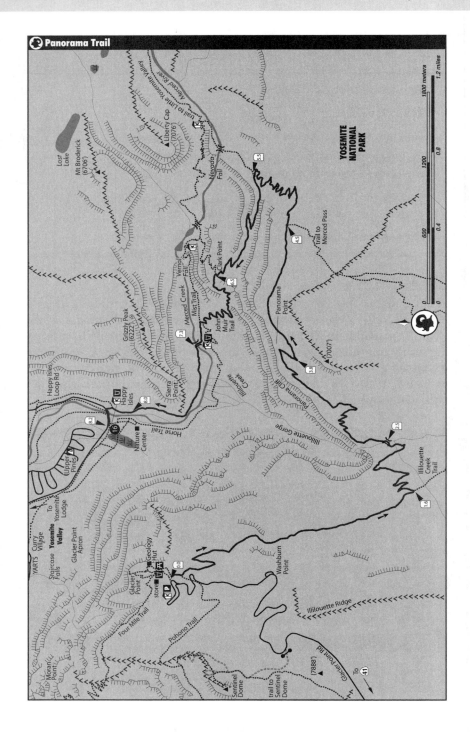

THE ROUTE

From the bus drop-off, head toward the large rock amphitheater to the east of the snack hut. The Panorama Trail begins atop a small slab just to the amphitheater's southwest—the starting point is signposted but unobtrusive. But first, if you have never been to Glacier Point (Hike 15), take 15 minutes and an additional 0.5 mile to walk to the vista point, for it provides views of Yosemite Falls and Yosemite Valley that you will not see on your hike. Also enjoy your current view of Half Dome, for its sheer northwest face is now prominently displayed, while later you will stare at its steep, narrower western side, and then its broad southern wall—the peak's profile is remarkably different from each direction.

Your descent begins through a scrubby slope of chinquapin oaks, prickly mountain whitethorns, and burnt stumps, the current (and evolving) landscape created by destructive fires in 1990. Small conifers are beginning to regrow and will eventually shade out the tangle of shrubs. After two switchbacks you embark on a long south-trending, descending traverse. About a third of the way down, both the top of Illilouette Falls and the Panorama Trail climbing beyond Illilouette Creek become visible. Where you reach a junction (**1.6 miles from start**), you turn left and begin a series of switchbacks down to Illilouette Creek. Near the end you reenter forest cover and twice step across a small tributary—likely dry by mid-season—and reach a handsome wooden bridge across the river (**2.5 miles**). (If you wish to swim, do so only when water levels are low. Head well upstream of the bridge, for the river rocks are well polished and dangerous. It is all too easy to lose your footing, even when the water is low, and slip into the stream and over a waterfall.)

Beyond the bridge you begin a steady climb—and by afternoon a hot one, for there is little shade and the sun will be beating from the southwest. A few spur trails to the left provide excellent views of Illilouette Falls. Indeed, at the top of the slope, the trail bypasses the point marked as Panorama Point on the USGS maps, but be cautious, as no railings exist to mark the edge. With effort, you ascend to the top of Panorama Cliff (**3.8 miles**). You now skirt along its top, climbing a few more switchbacks in a patch of forest but generally continuing eastward along a mostly open, quite certainly panoramic trail. Please avoid the temptation to push rocks or logs off the cliff—as I saw someone doing when I last passed here—for in stretches, the John Muir Trail is exactly at the base of this escarpment.

Your descent resumes beyond a junction (**4.5 miles**). Here you turn left and descend shaded switchbacks to the top of Nevada Fall, while the right-hand choice leads eventually to Merced Pass. The trail here is pleasant walking—a few rocks to step around but soft forest floor on which to walk. In spring you will be delighted by patches of western azaleas covered with large, light pink flowers. The last stretch of the descent is on slab; note the low rock walls once built to divert runoff away from the cliff face and the unseen trail below.

Your next junction is with the John Muir Trail, and you now turn left to begin the descent alongside Nevada Fall **(5.5 miles)**; heading right would take you to the Merced River at the top of Nevada Fall and beyond to Half Dome. Traversing a walled ledge, you have fantastic views of the waterfall and the domes behind—Half Dome lies behind Mount Broderick and Liberty Cap. Beyond the ledge, long switchbacks resume, with views of the domes each time you reach the eastward side of a zigzag. These take you to another junction, Clark Point **(6.5 miles)**.

The John Muir Trail continues to the left, while right is a connector trail leading to the Mist Trail above Vernal Fall. You head left, first along a gently slanting slope and then sneaking into a gully that lies directly beneath Panorama Cliff. Indeed, this gully is the only break in the cliff

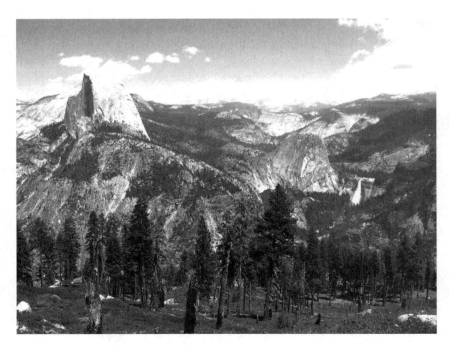

Half Dome, Liberty Cap, and Nevada Fall

face—from Glacier Point to Nevada Fall—and therefore the only location where you can easily reach the valley floor. (The Mist Trail of course descends as well, but the trail follows a thin, fenced ledge.) Endless switchbacks ensue, and I always find them tough on the feet at the end of a hike because long stretches are paved with granite cobble to avoid trail erosion. Shortly after the slope becomes shallower, you first pass a horse trail and then reach a T-junction with the Mist Trail. Here you turn left and within minutes you reach the bridge, restrooms, water fountain, and large number of people at the base of Vernal Fall **(7.3 miles)**.

Halfway across the large bridge, stop and enjoy the view of Vernal Fall; the afternoon lighting is wonderful. Continuing to the far end of the bridge, follow the now-paved trail the last stretch to the valley floor. Stop and enjoy the vista where the trail turns to the right, for here you can look up to Glacier Point, your starting point many hours ago. Once at the trailhead **(8.0 miles)**, continue straight ahead along the river's east bank until you reach the road. Turn left, cross the bridge, and you will be at the shuttle stop **(8.2 miles)**.

TO THE TRAILHEAD

GPS Coordinates:
Glacier Point parking lot: N37° 43.661' W119° 34.462'
Happy Isles shuttle stop: N37° 43.976' W119° 36.070'
If you plan to do a car shuttle or have someone drop you at Glacier Point, see Glacier Point (Hike 15) for driving directions. A logistically easier alternative is to take a tour bus from Yosemite Lodge to Glacier Point. (See the Glacier Point tour link at **nps.gov/yose/planyourvisit/bus.htm** for information on buses.) At the end of the day you will take the Yosemite Valley shuttle bus from Happy Isles back to your car, campground, or lodging.

Park your car at your Yosemite Valley accommodation or at the large Yosemite Village visitor parking lot (shuttle stop 1) and take the Valley shuttle to Yosemite Lodge (stop 8). If you are driving from outside the valley, to reach the parking lot, drive east (toward Half Dome) on Southside Drive until you reach Sentinel Bridge, 4.1 miles from where CA 41 merges with Valley Loop Road and your first stop sign. Straight ahead takes you to Curry Village, while turning left takes you across Sentinel Bridge to Yosemite Village and Yosemite Lodge. Turn left and after 0.3 mile you reach a second stop sign; turning left takes you to Yosemite Lodge, while you turn right to Yosemite Village. Continue east for 0.1 mile to another stop sign and turn right into a large dirt parking area.

18 Lower Chilnualna Falls

Trailhead Location: Northeast end of Wawona residential area

Trail Use: Hiking

Distance & Configuration: 0.7-mile out-and-back

Elevation Range: 4,150 feet at the start, with 300 feet of ascent/descent

Facilities: Toilets are present at the trailhead. Water is available at the Wawona Store.

Highlights: A tangle of gushing cascades and fractured granite blocks, as well as old rock walls

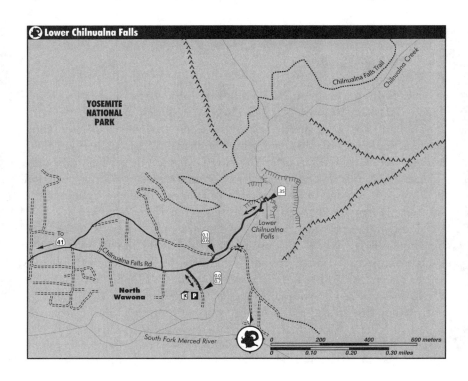

DESCRIPTION

In spring and early summer lower Chilnualna Falls is a collection of many churning 15- to 30-foot waterfalls flowing along fractures in steep granite walls. The walk is up the old trail, now for foot use only and featuring elegant rock walls. This walk is accessible year-round but best seen May–July for the waterfalls.

THE ROUTE

From the parking area, return to the road on which you drove in, turn right, and continue 300 feet until a sign indicates that this is not a through street. Signs now direct you up a steep road on your left. As you turn and begin ascending this road, almost immediately note a small trail departing on the right **(0.1 mile from start)**. This is the footpath, while horses are required to continue up the road to a second trailhead. (The two trails reunite 0.4 mile ahead, along the trail to upper Chilnualna Falls and beyond your destination.)

Take the foot trail, which traverses a steep slope above boulder-filled Chilnualna Creek. Passing through a diverse forest that includes incense cedars, black oaks, white firs, and live oaks, the trail ascends, maintaining its elevation above the tumbling creek. In places the grade is unusually steep for a Sierra trail, while elsewhere switchbacks lined by beautiful, old, mossy rock walls ease the ascent. Ahead you see the first and tallest of the cascades dropping into a beautiful pool, perfect for a midsummer dip—but only be tempted to swim when the water levels are low. A giant boulder just downstream provides an excellent vista location.

While most people turn around at this point, I encourage you to continue a short stretch farther until the trail turns resolutely left and away from the drainage **(0.35 mile)**. Ahead are many more cascades, as the water weaves among the many fractures in the blocky, jointed rock. A few small rock spires ascend above the water. Western azalea bushes that line sections of shore are colorful in spring. Return the way you came **(0.7 mile)**.

TO THE TRAILHEAD

GPS Coordinates: N37° 32.853' W119° 38.067'
Head to the location in Yosemite Valley where Southside Drive, the eastbound road in the valley, and CA 41, the road from Wawona, meet. If you are in Yosemite Village or Curry Village, this requires taking westbound

Northside Drive to the western end of the valley. Stay in the left lane to cross the Merced River. After 0.9 mile you will reach the CA 41 junction and turn right onto CA 41. Continue along CA 41 for 21.3 miles, passing through the Wawona Tunnel, past Glacier Point Road (at Chinquapin), and many turns later reaching the first road in Wawona, Chilnualna Falls Road. (The Wawona Store is an additional 0.2 mile along CA 41, at the intersection with Forest Drive.) Turn left and drive 1.9 miles to nearly the end of Chilnualna Falls Road, passing through an extensive residential area before reaching a dirt parking area on your right; park here. The trailhead is just beyond to the left of the road. (Wawona is 20.6 miles north of Oakhurst.)

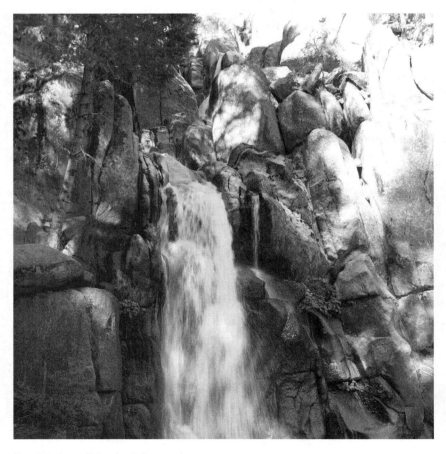

One of the lower Chilnualna Falls cascades

19 Wawona Meadow

Trailhead Location: Wawona

Trail Use: Hiking

Distance & Configuration: 3.6-mile loop

Elevation Range: 4,000 feet at the start, with a cumulative elevation change of ±220 feet

Facilities: Toilets and water are available at the Wawona Store.

Highlights: Magnificent spring wildflowers, split log fences, and Wawona Hotel

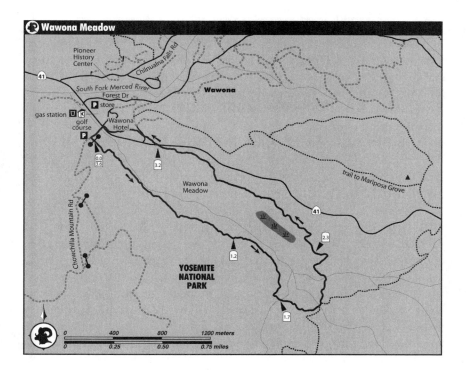

DESCRIPTION

The quiet, nearly flat walk around Wawona Meadow is a perfect selection for enjoying spring wildflowers or for a winter walk when most locations are snow covered. The split rail fence surrounding the meadow makes a beautiful foreground.

THE ROUTE

Heading south along the locked fire road, you are beginning your circumnavigation of Wawona Meadow. As you will quickly discover, the trail's name, Wawona Meadow Loop, is a misnomer, for you never actually enter the quite marshy Wawona Meadow and mostly see it only from afar, instead keeping to the forest encircling the meadow. It is a forest dominated by red-barked incense cedars, with white firs and ponderosa pines mixed in. The deciduous black oaks grow along the meadow's edge. Deer are often present along the meadow's edge, especially late in the day. In spring and into summer wildflowers are abundant, and there are even patches of wild strawberries to entice children. A split log fence, recently restored, lies between the meadow and the road, reminding you of Wawona's pioneer past.

The road has climbed gently since the start, but only after it turns to a more southerly trajectory does it begin to feel uphill **(1.2 miles from start)**. Shortly it reaches the first of three creek crossings, one of the three forks of the unnamed tributary of the South Fork of the Merced River that run through the middle of Wawona Meadow **(1.7 miles)**. Soon you reach the southern end of the meadow and a moister bit of forest, decorated in spring by the mountain dogwood's large white flowers and in fall by its colored leaves. Forest openings allow you glimpses of Wawona Dome to the northeast. You step across a second creek and in quick succession pass two unmarked trail junctions; stay left at each of them.

You step across a third creek, either on stones or a small log if the water flows are high. Now on the warmer side of the meadow, you find yourself passing colorful fields of wildflowers, especially noting sections of dry meadow blanketed with clarkia, with its large two-toned pink flowers. Carpets of strong-smelling mountain misery grow beneath scattered trees. You are now, for the first time, right at the meadow's edge and can enjoy verdant green grass and scattered willows **(2.3 miles)**. Flowers are plentiful at the trail's edge, and the log fence still divides you from the main meadow. Birds are abundant, enjoying the meadow's insect life. You are now nearly parallel to the main road and slowly converge with it as you continue around the meadow.

The approaching golf course marks the end of your quiet meadow walk, for now you cross the main road **(3.2 miles)**, walk a short stretch along a sandy trail, and merge with a paved road that skirts around the back of the Wawona Hotel. Before you reach the back of the hotel, a small trail cuts left off the paved road. Follow this trail around to the front of the hotel; if you find yourself around the back side of buildings, you have gone too far. Stop in front of the magnificent Victorian hotel, built in 1876, before crossing the main road and walking up the spur road to your car **(3.6 miles)**.

TO THE TRAILHEAD

GPS Coordinates: N37° 32.100' W119° 39.450'

Head to the location in Yosemite Valley where Southside Drive, the eastbound road in the valley, and CA 41, the road from Wawona, meet. If you are in Yosemite Village or Curry Village, this requires taking westbound Northside Drive to the western end of the valley. Stay in the left lane to cross the Merced River. After 0.9 mile you will reach the CA 41 junction and turn right onto CA 41. Continue along CA 41 for 21.5 miles, passing through the Wawona Tunnel and past Glacier Point Road before reaching the Wawona Store. Next, 0.3 mile beyond the store, turn right onto the spur road across the street from the Wawona Hotel. Continue 0.1 mile to the west side of the meadow, where you will see a closed road—the trail—heading south; park along the side of the road.

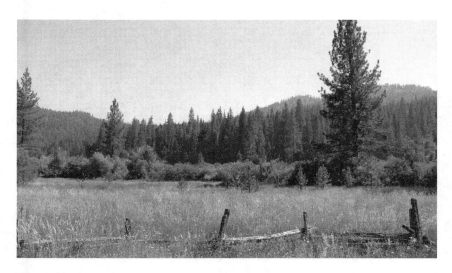

Wawona Meadow

20 Mariposa Grove

Trailhead Location: Mariposa Grove, south of Wawona

Trail Use: Hiking

Distance & Configuration: 4.9-mile loop

Elevation Range: 5,620 feet at the start, with a cumulative elevation change of ±1,040 feet

Facilities: Water and a snack bar are located at the trailhead shuttle stop, while a large toilet block is just to the left (north) at the entrance to the parking lot. Water and toilets are also present at the museum in the Upper Grove.

Highlights: Two large groves of giant sequoias, majestic trunks, and remembering why Yosemite exists

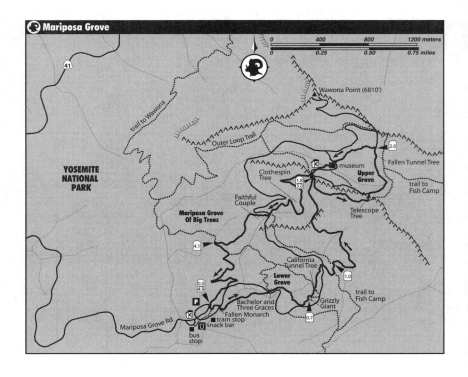

DESCRIPTION

The Upper and Lower Mariposa Groves are the two largest stands of sequoias in Yosemite. An equally important reason for a visit is to read and think about the historical importance of this grove. It is one of the reasons the national park was created and was home to Yosemite's first guardian, Galen Clark. The Mariposa Grove is snow covered in winter and only accessible by snowshoes or skis.

THE ROUTE

Upon arriving at the shuttle stop (or parking lot), you will notice the majority of people heading for a ticket counter, procuring a ride on a large open-air tram. Some people ride just to the top and walk down, while most ride the complete loop. The option is tempting, especially on a hot summer day, but I encourage you to think twice about walking both directions. Sequoia trees are overwhelming in size, yet majestic, and you cannot truly absorb their splendor while wearing a pair of headphones and sitting on a vehicle a considerable distance from the trees. And it is while heading uphill that you walk slowly and stop and stare at your surroundings.

The trailhead is at the back right corner of the parking area. If you arrive by shuttle, to reach the trailhead, pass the snack bar and continue on a trail that skirts the right (south) side of the parking lot. Pick up one of the small trail brochures to read about the natural and human history of the Mariposa Grove, but note that in a recent edition several errors were in the map. When in doubt follow the signs on the trail, not the map. Turning right you immediately reach the first landmark, the Fallen Monarch, a large tree that fell long before Galen Clark recorded the grove in 1857.

Continuing along the trail you immediately cross a swampy area on a bridge and next cross the tram road before beginning a climb across the base of a bare slope. The slope to the right has been severely burnt, but the fire does little damage to the sequoia trees. Their bark is so thick (2 feet!) and fire resistant that they are not killed by fire. Indeed their seedlings depend upon it, requiring bare soil and sunshine to germinate. Walking up newly built steps and crossing the tram road again, you next pass a cluster of trees named the Bachelor and the Three Graces. Above you walk through a lovely shaded stretch, often a little muddy to the sides as you cross small trickles. The next destination is the Grizzly Giant, one of the grove's largest trees **(0.7 mile from start)**. It is set behind a wooden fence to protect its delicate roots, for despite their great size, sequoia roots are quite close to the surface and easily disturbed. Stop and stare at these beautiful trees. Admire their girth, stately trunks, and unusual branch architecture.

Encircling the Grizzly Giant to the left, you come to an X-junction where you continue straight ahead, right through the center of the California Tunnel Tree and on up to another crossing of the tram road. Just above you reach a junction where you turn left (right leads to Fish Camp) and immediately reach a second junction (1.0 mile), where you stay right. Families with young children may decide to end their walk here and retrace their steps downhill. You have now left the Lower Grove and are beginning a traverse through open fir forest to the Upper Grove. The dry, steep slope you ascend is not suitable sequoia habitat, and on a hot afternoon many a hiker is wishing for a little more shade and a lower angle slope. At the top of the slope you reach a five-way junction and take a sharp right-hand turn toward the Telescope Tree (1.8 miles).

The trail leads east up the crest of a shallow ridge, with sequoias to your left and burnt fir trees on the right. A sign eventually points left to the Telescope Tree. Head a short distance downhill to stare up at the sky through the hole in the center of the tree. You could now retrace your steps to the trail, but I recommend walking along the tram road for a short stretch, for you pass a lovely grove of midsize sequoias in a flower-filled meadow and then reach the famous fallen Wawona Tunnel Tree. The tunnel was carved out in 1881 and countless people and vehicles drove through it for 88 years before the tree fell in the winter of 1969. Just beyond the Wawona Tunnel Tree, turn left onto a trail descending toward the museum (2.6 miles).

Descending steeply along a sunnier stretch of slope, you pass a collection of young trees, cross the tram road again, and reach the museum, a cabin that was built in 1930 at the site of Galen Clark's 1864 cabin. The grove of trees below the museum is one of my favorites, framed in early summer by a thicket of yellow-flowered, arrow-leaved groundsel that contrasts wonderfully against the red-brown trunks. As you descend, stay left at the first junction, pass toilets, and reach the same five-way junction as before (3.0 miles). Now head straight downhill on the trail, signposted for the Clothespin Tree. You pass the tree and cross the tram road yet again, continuing straight ahead. (At this point an unmarked trail departs to the left—southeast; stay straight.) Next you pass the Faithful Couple, two trees whose trunks have merged together, and continue down.

Reaching a T-junction, you turn left (right is the Outer Loop Trail that heads toward Wawona and also back to the Upper Grove) (4.1 miles), and then head right at a second junction. You now switchback down the final stretch to the trailhead (4.9 miles) and retrace your steps to your car or the shuttle stop.

TO THE TRAILHEAD

GPS Coordinates: N37° 30.144' W119° 36.583'

Head to the location in Yosemite Valley where Southside Drive, the east-bound road in the valley, and CA 41, the road from Wawona, meet. If you are in Yosemite Village or Curry Village, this requires taking westbound Northside Drive to the western end of the valley. Stay in the left lane to cross the Merced River. After 0.9 mile you will reach the CA 41 junction and turn right onto CA 41. Continue along CA 41 for 21.5 miles, passing through the Wawona Tunnel and past Glacier Point Road before reaching the Wawona Store. Continue south on CA 41 for an additional 4.7 miles to reach Mariposa Grove Road (just before the park exit station). Turn left and drive 4.6 miles to the end of Mariposa Grove Road.

Note that if the parking lot at the end of this road is full, you must park either in a small lot at the junction of CA 41 and Mariposa Grove Road or at the Wawona Store parking area, and take a shuttle bus to the trailhead. If you are arriving after early morning, you should park at the Wawona Store and take the shuttle to avoid being turned back.

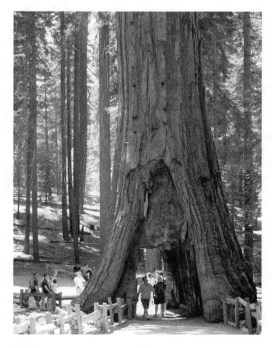

Walking through the California Tunnel Tree

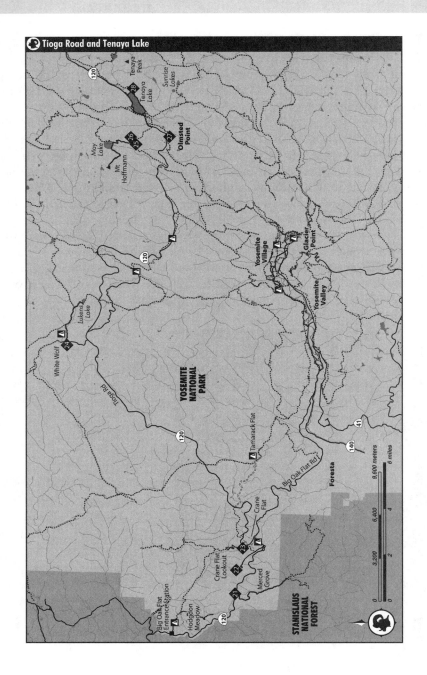

TIOGA ROAD AND TENAYA LAKE

Regional Overview

This region's trailheads extend across 3,000 feet of elevation and along 36 miles of CA 120, Tioga Road, from the Merced Grove to Tenaya Lake. Much of this distance is through Yosemite's diverse mid-elevation conifer forests, bisected by many creeks and dotted with meadows. At the western end are two of Yosemite's groves of giant sequoias, and at the eastern end is Tenaya Lake, marking the beginning of the high country.

The hikes reflect this large geographic extent and accompanying diversity and include visits to the sequoia groves (Merced Grove, Hike 21, and Tuolumne Grove, Hike 23), a visit to a historic fire tower (Hike 22), walks through quiet conifer forests to lakes and along streams (Lukens Lake, Hike 24, and May Lake, Hike 25), two walks that accentuate the granite slabs of the Tenaya Lake area (Olmsted Point, Hike 27, and Tenaya Lake, Hike 28), and a walk to a summit at the geographical center of Yosemite (Mount Hoffmann, Hike 26). During early to mid-July, when the flowers are at their peak, the forest and stream bank walks that define this region are wonderfully beautiful and engaging (and often swarming with mosquitoes). If you have come to Yosemite for big views and lots of rock instead, climb Mount Hoffmann, or continue east to Tuolumne Meadows and Tioga Pass to emerge from forest cover.

Parents walking with children will likely select the walks with instant gratification. The quick jaunts to the Crane Flat fire tower (Hike 22) or Olmsted Point (Hike 27) are recommended quick stops to break up a drive and get everyone out of the car for 30 minutes. Anyone who can walk can complete these and will enjoy the endpoint. A walk around Tenaya Lake (Hike 28) is also a fantastic walk with young children, for it is a flat walk with a beautiful lake and swimming beaches. A child older than age 5 can easily walk to the Tuolumne Grove (Hike 23), but remember that it is a steep climb out. May Lake (Hike 25) is an easy walk to an exquisite lake, but make sure that everyone knows about the no-swimming regulation before you begin to avoid disappointment. An 8-year-old (or older child) would thoroughly enjoy the accolades received while climbing Mount Hoffmann (Hike 26), but this is a long climb. The remaining hikes are less recommended for children unless your child is one who can easily be propelled forward by wildflower or pinecone hunts.

Note that Hikes 24–28 are accessed from Tioga Road, open approximately Memorial Day–late October. Be sure to check the Yosemite National Park website for opening and closing dates, as they are determined by that year's snowpack. And it is usually mid-June or early July before sufficient snow has melted to actually take these walks.

◘ ◘ ◘

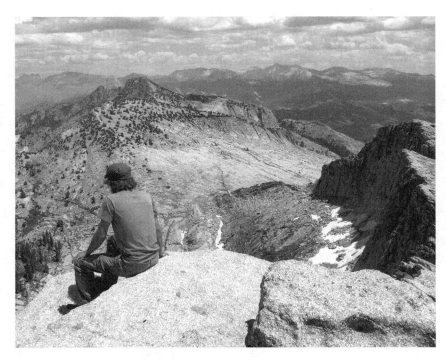

Looking northeast from the summit of Mount Hoffmann (see page 125)

21 Merced Grove

Trailhead Location: CA 120, west of Crane Flat

Trail Use: Hiking

Distance & Configuration: 3.2-mile out-and-back

Elevation Range: 5,860 feet at the start, with 500 feet of descent/ascent

Facilities: A toilet is at the parking area, and picnic tables are just west of the trailhead. The closest water is at the Crane Flat Store at the T-junction at Crane Flat.

Highlights: Giant sequoias all to yourself and a row of six large red "elephant feet"

DESCRIPTION

The smallest of Yosemite's three giant sequoia groves, the Merced Grove is also the quietest. Even midsummer you will see only a few people as you descend an old road to two clusters of large trees, including six giants in a near-perfect line.

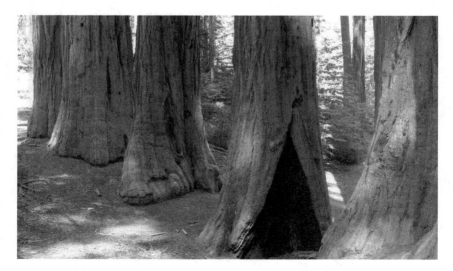

A row of giant sequoias

THE ROUTE

Leaving the parking area you skirt around a locked gate and amble along a fire trail. This was the first road into Yosemite Valley, Coulterville Road, descending past the Merced Grove before contouring around slopes en route to the community of Foresta. It is now a remarkably quiet location, allowing you to enjoy the forest sounds and smells without the chatter of Yosemite's many visitors. The dirt road is pleasant walking, for there is initially little elevation change. Walking in and out of dense forest cover, note that the slopes above you tend to be shallower, sunnier, and dry, while dense conifer forests dominate on the steep shaded slopes deeper into the drainage. The giant sequoias you will soon see might be the biggest trees, but this stretch of forest includes some impressive specimens of

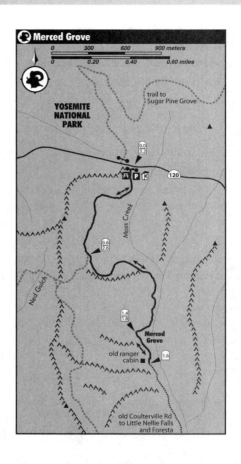

other species: sugar pines, with their gigantic cones, and the smaller-coned western white pines. At a Y-junction, head left, beginning your descent into the canyon **(0.6 mile from start)**.

The trail now descends more steeply to Moss Creek. The air temperature feels cooler and moister as you descend the north and then east-facing slopes—this is the climate preferred by the giant sequoias. In the draw are mountain dogwoods and hazelnuts, while wild roses, the tall stalks of pinedrops, and small orchids grow adjacent to the trail. Soon you reach the banks of Moss Creek and parallel it downstream. Where the trail diverges slightly from the creek, you round a corner and are greeted by six sequoias growing in a remarkably straight line **(1.4 miles)**. Their bases remind me of red, shaggy elephant feet, impressively massive and slightly larger than the sturdy trunks above. Here, unlike the more visited groves, the trail takes you close to the trees, allowing you to absorb their full grandeur, but be aware that their shallow roots are damaged by human footsteps and respect signs asking you to stick to the trail.

Continuing on, you reach additional trees, including both the largest in the Merced Grove and some young trees **(1.6 miles)**. Notice how thick their bark is. These trees can easily withstand fire and indeed require a fire-cleared landscape for seeds to germinate. Nestled among this lower group of sequoias is an old ranger's cabin as well as a bench for a quiet, secluded rest before beginning the climb back away from the creek. (The fire road now ends and only a narrow trail continues downstream. If you wish to continue farther, there are a few more sequoias.) Return to your car the way you came **(3.2 miles)**.

TO THE TRAILHEAD

GPS Coordinates: N37° 45.780' W119° 50.535'

From the CA 120 entrance station (the Big Oak Flat entrance station), drive 3.7 miles east on CA 120. The parking area is on your right as you come to the crest of a long hill. (This location is 4 miles west of the T-junction at Crane Flat, where CA 120 from Tuolumne Meadows and Big Oak Flat Road from Yosemite Valley intersect.)

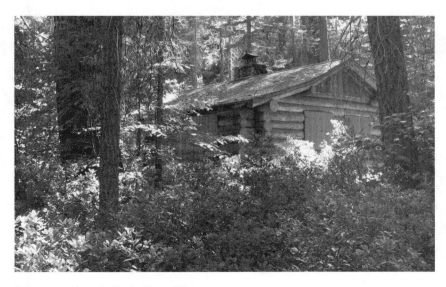

Old ranger cabin tucked in the Merced Grove

22 Crane Flat Lookout

Trailhead Location: CA 120, west of Crane Flat

Trail Use: Hiking

Distance & Configuration: 0.4-mile out-and-back

Elevation Range: 6,605 feet at the start, with 40 feet of ascent/descent

Facilities: No amenities are at the trailhead, but toilets are available at the lookout. The closest water is at the Crane Flat Store.

Highlights: Historic fire tower and distant views of the Dardanelles and the Clark Range

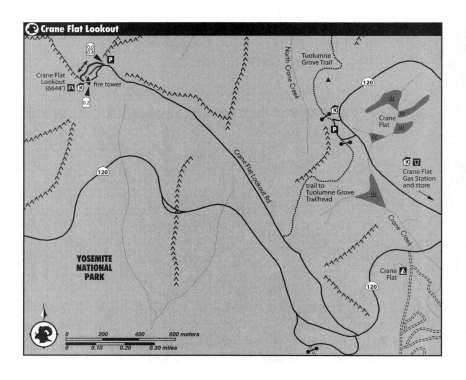

DESCRIPTION

The historic Crane Flat Fire Station is open to visitors and accessible by a very short walk. From the tower you will enjoy impressive views of western Yosemite and get a feel for the expansive forests constantly being monitored for new fire activity.

THE ROUTE

Standing in the dirt parking area with the helipad to your left, you are facing a tall wall of bushes—bitter cherry and mountain whitethorn. The barricade of prickles is broken by a small, signed trail and, during recent summers, a bulletin board with current Yosemite fire information. The narrow trail begins a remarkably long loop to the west of the helipad, mostly flanked by chokecherry too tall to see over. A few indistinct paths depart to the right. When in doubt, stay to the left.

When you emerge from the bushes, you see a toilet and picnic table to your right and the fire tower ahead **(0.2 mile from start)**. The fire tower, built in 1931 and on the National Register of Historic Places, is

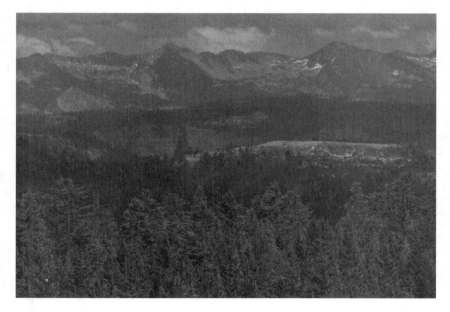

View to the Clark Range from the lookout

still in use. Signs welcome you up to the observation deck. You can both walk around the outside enjoying views of the surrounding peaks and walk inside to see the equipment used by the fire spotters and sign your name in the logbook. To the northwest you can see the Dardanelles, dark volcanic mesas and spires; to the northeast is Tower Peak; and to the east is Mount Lyell, Yosemite's high point, and the Clark Range. In between are miles and miles of forest that can be observed from this location. Enjoy the view and return to the car the way you came **(0.4 mile)**.

In winter the fire lookout can be accessed on skis or snowshoes from Crane Flat. Park at the Tuolumne Grove parking area and follow the yellow ski markers, but note that this short walk then becomes a 3.0-mile trip.

TO THE TRAILHEAD
GPS Coordinates: N37° 45.636' W119° 49.176'
From the CA 120 entrance station (the Big Oak Flat entrance station), drive 6.9 miles east on CA 120. A sign indicates the Crane Flat lookout on the north (left) side of the road. Drive up this paved road 1.4 miles to a parking lot at its end. Note that this road may be closed to vehicles during periods of fire danger or during fire operations. (This location is 0.8 mile west of the T-junction at Crane Flat, where CA 120 from Tuolumne Meadows and Big Oak Flat Road from Yosemite Valley intersect.)

23 Tuolumne Grove

Trailhead Location: Crane Flat

Trail Use: Hiking, stroller accessible but steep

Distance & Configuration: 2.7-mile out-and-back

Elevation Range: 6,190 feet at the start, with a cumulative elevation change of ±500 feet

Facilities: Toilets are located at the trailhead, but the closest water is at the Crane Flat Store.

Highlights: Giant sequoias, cones of giant sugar pines, and dogwoods blooming in spring

DESCRIPTION

If you have time to visit only one of Yosemite's giant sequoia groves, make it the Tuolumne Grove. Although smaller than the Mariposa Grove, this grove also boasts a tunnel tree, fallen trees with exquisite roots, several clusters of beautiful living trees, and excellent information placards. And it is a much quieter location with far fewer people and no trams—simply a pleasant walk through forest and past giant sugar pine cones to the grove. For families with young children, a particular attraction of this walk is that for most of the distance you are walking along a paved road along which you are permitted to push a stroller.

THE ROUTE

The paved trail departs from the west end of the parking lot, adjacent to a display of a large tree slice. It is a stretch of the original CA 120 and continued to be accessible to one-way traffic (from Hodgdon Meadow) until 1993. The route traverses across and down a steep forested slope as it descends toward the big trees. In spring the white blossoms of the mountain dogwoods and scattered low-growing pink roses decorate the walk. The attentive visitor might also catch a glimpse of wild orchids along the road banks. While most plants at this elevation bloom in spring, a giant patch of coneflowers blooms in August and is impossible to miss as you round a corner to the left **(0.3 mile from start)**.

The descent continues, first with a northward trajectory and then south, all the while under a mixed conifer canopy of incense cedars, white firs,

Douglas firs, and sugar pines. Soon after you turn back to the north, you pass a sign indicating that you are entering the grove **(1.0 mile)**. The giant sequoias were once more widely distributed in the Sierra, but today appropriate climatic conditions generally exist only in open draws between elevations of 4,000 and 6,000 feet. The first trees are now visible in the forest to the left (west) of the trail, but walk until the trail curves to the right to begin gawking at these stout giants. The girth of their trunks is the most impressive, but also stare at their robust branches and rounded canopy. The giant sequoias have such a different form than the intermingled pines and firs. Around your feet you may notice pinecones that exceed a foot in length. These belong to the co-occurring sugar pines; the sequoia cones are less than an inch long.

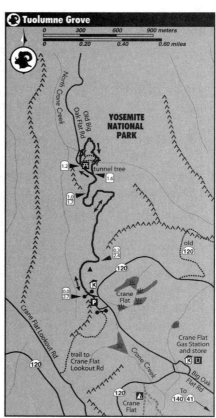

Opposite the first large sequoia, you will note a trail junction to your right (north); this is the route by which you will return. For now continue down the road to an opening with picnic tables and information placards **(1.2 miles)**. Many trails depart from this location; select the trail to the far left (west) that is lined with a hewn log fence and follows the banks of a small creek. (If you are pushing a stroller, you will now need to return the way you came or leave your stroller here to retrieve later.)

This loop trail will take you past several fallen trees as well as a grove of young individuals, eventually leading to an opening where you can admire the upended roots of a large tree. From this location, your route heads left around the top of these roots, steps across two small creeks on wooden bridges, and shortly reaches a famous tunnel tree. A long-ago fire shaped its cathedral-like form. The wood is so resistant to decay that it maintains this form centuries after the fire. Turn left and walk up through the tunnel, enjoying its skylight. After a brief ascent, you descend to the paved road near the first of the sequoias you admired earlier **(1.6 miles)**. Where you merge with the paved road, turn left (uphill) and retrace your steps to the parking area **(2.7 miles)**.

TO THE TRAILHEAD
GPS Coordinates: N37° 45.496' W119° 48.329'
Big Oak Flat Road from Yosemite Valley and CA 120 intersect at a T-junction in Crane Flat. Turn north at this T-junction, toward Tuolumne Meadows. After 0.6 mile turn left into a large parking area. (Crane Flat is located 7.7 miles east of the CA 120 entrance station, 23.7 miles northwest of Yosemite Village, and 39.4 miles west of the Tuolumne Meadows Store.)

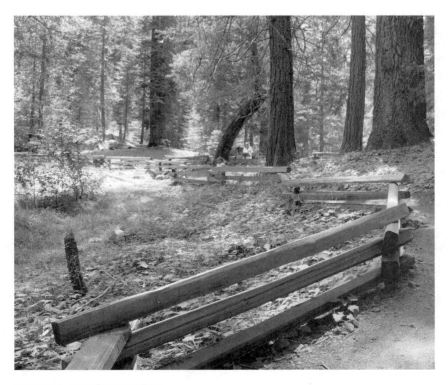

A walk through the Tuolumne Grove

24 Lukens Lake (from White Wolf)

Trailhead Location: White Wolf, north of Tioga Road

Trail Use: Hiking

Distance & Configuration: 4.6-mile out-and-back

Elevation Range: 7,875 feet at the start, with a cumulative elevation change of ±380 feet

Facilities: Water and toilets are available at the trailhead. Snacks are for sale at the north end of the High Sierra Camp dining tent.

Highlights: Expanses of wildflowers, bright bursts of color, and a quiet lake

DESCRIPTION

The walk to Lukens Lake is exquisite during the wildflower season, usually June–mid-July, for the trail takes you past one lush, forest-ringed meadow after another, each a blanket of flowers. The creek banks are equally colorful, decorated with tall, colorful stalks. The expansive meadows at the southeast end of Lukens Lake are the final highlight, where you can enjoy concentric rings of color, each indicating a different species growing an increasing distance from the lakeshore.

THE ROUTE

Departing from the northeast end of the parking lot, the trail skirts the south side of the White Wolf Campground and continues through dense lodgepole pine forest. This first stretch of the walk is along a wide, nearly flat trail, and you can walk quite quickly, passing some giant boulders and enjoying the bright green understory, before long reaching a crossing of the Middle Tuolumne River **(0.6 mile from start)**. You can currently cross the creek on a large downed log, but when this log disappears, it will be a sandy-bottomed wade when water levels are high. At the next junction **(0.8 mile)**, turn right and continue your walk through an unusually lush forest of lodgepole pines and red firs. You now begin to pass meadow upon meadow, all brightly colored with flowers in spring and summer and shifting to an equally rich yellow by fall. Especially prevalent in the marshiest areas are expanses of lilac shooting stars and tall, white-flowered corn

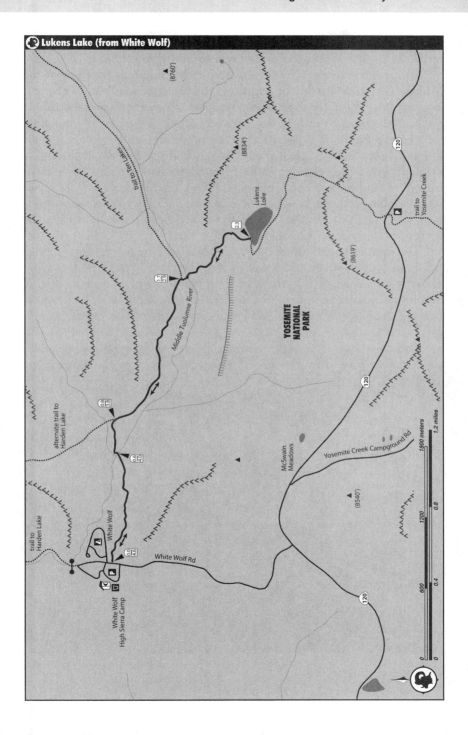

Lukens Lake (from White Wolf)

lilies. Note that mosquitoes can be just as abundant as the flowers. Between meadows the flowers are sparser but still adorn the forest floor.

At the next junction **(1.7 miles)**, keep right and immediately cross the Middle Tuolumne River a second time, this time on a collection of small logs, or possibly if the logs have disappeared, another sandy-bottomed wade. The stream bank here explodes with color, a preview of your final flower-lined ascent to Lukens Lake. You now climb to the left of a shallow gully, through which just enough water drains to create a slope densely planted with tall flowers; alpine lilies, groundsels, cow parsnips, geraniums, corn lilies, and more are intermingled. While the meadows were often an intense splash of a single color, these sloping meadows are a mixed bouquet. Climbing steadily, the trail bends to the right and shortly reaches the shores of Lukens Lake **(2.3 miles)**.

The shallow shores along the lake's northwest are perfect for a picnic, sitting in dappled shade and watching birds perched on the dead logs lying at the water's edge. Across the lake are more bursts of color from a large meadow, absolutely chock-full of flowers in early summer. Most impressive are the rings of color, as different species prefer the wetter soils in

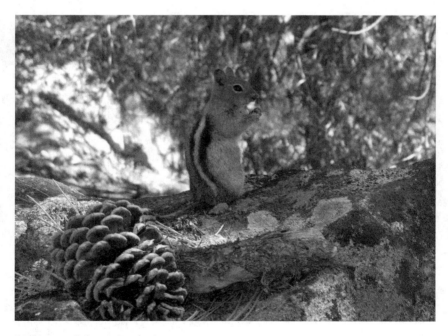

A golden-mantled ground squirrel

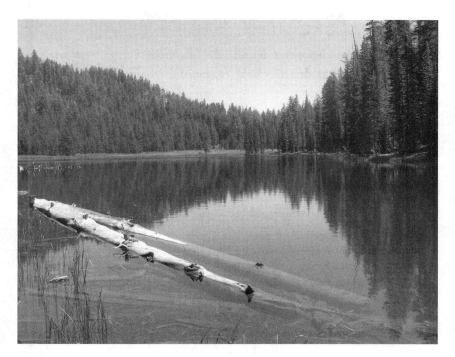

Lukens Lake

the middle and others require the drier soils near the meadow's edge. The meadow is currently a regeneration area and you are asked to admire it from afar. If your current view is unsatisfying, follow the trail to the lake's outlet and along the southern shore for a closer view. Return to White Wolf the way you came **(4.6 miles)**.

TO THE TRAILHEAD
GPS Coordinates: N37° 52.194' W119° 38.926'
Big Oak Flat Road from Yosemite Valley and CA 120 intersect at a T-junction in Crane Flat. Turn north at this T-junction, toward Tuolumne Meadows. After 14.5 miles turn left onto White Wolf Road. Drive 1.1 miles down White Wolf Road to a parking area. (Crane Flat is located 7.7 miles east of the CA 120 entrance station and 23.7 miles northwest of Yosemite Village.) Alternatively, drive 24.9 miles west from the Tuolumne Meadows Store on CA 120.

25 May Lake

Trailhead Location: May Lake Trailhead, 2 miles north of Tioga Road

Trail Use: Hiking

Distance & Configuration: 2.9-mile out-and-back

Elevation Range: 8,845 feet at the start, with 500 feet of ascent/descent

Facilities: Toilets are at the trailhead. Drinking water and toilets are available at the May Lake Campground, 1.1 miles into this hike, and at locations in Tuolumne Meadows, the White Wolf High Sierra Camp, and the Crane Flat Store.

Highlights: Granite slab–ringed lake, endless undulating granite ridges, and hemlock groves

DESCRIPTION

The view from the hemlock-ringed banks of May Lake is stark and impressive: steep, smooth granite slabs above a deep, dark-blue lake. It is a worthwhile picnic spot even though swimming is not permitted. A short detour onto granite slabs east of the lake is one of the best locations to absorb the vastness of the granite slabs around Tenaya Lake and the Cathedral Range. Note that the spur road to May Lake often opens several weeks after Tioga Road.

THE ROUTE

Adjacent to the trailhead is a boggy tarn, home to a large population of mosquitoes, so organize your backpacks quickly and don't be deterred from going on this walk. These are the worst bugs you will encounter, for May Lake mostly lacks the shallow bays that the mosquitoes love.

Looping around the tarn, the trail begins its route northward to May Lake. You climb slowly through an open forest, passing many small outcrops and patches of granite slab. The bedrock laid bare by glaciers lies not far below the surface; in some places sufficient soil exists to support sparse tree and shrub cover, and elsewhere the rock slab slopes too much for soil to accumulate. Breaks in tree cover allow views east to the Cathedral Range and south to Clouds Rest and Half Dome. To ascend a steeper

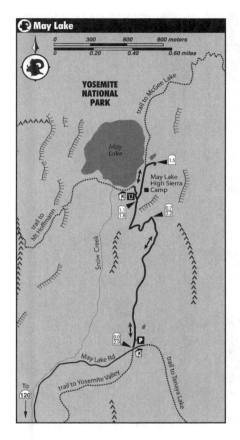

slope **(0.7 mile from start)**, the trail switchbacks a few times and trends a little to the west before again turning north.

This climb takes you to a flat of mountain hemlocks and western white pines and after a few steps to a marked junction, a toilet, and a drinking water tap **(1.1 miles)**. Straight ahead takes you to the May Lake High Sierra Camp, while left takes you to the backpacker campground, the picturesque south shore of the lake, and the trail to Mount Hoffmann (Hike 26). Take this left-hand fork, for it quickly leads to the shoreline as well as many locations to sit on a boulder or fallen log and stare out over the expanse of blue water, which is ringed to the north and west by granite slabs. And although swimming is prohibited, fishing is permitted.

Afterward, I recommend retracing your steps to the junction **(1.2 miles)**. Now head straight ahead, passing through the middle of the High Sierra Camp. After 0.2 mile you reach a point where May Lake's shoreline juts a little to the east, and there is a tarn to the east of the trail. At this point, skirt around the southern edge of the tarn and scramble onto the slab ridge to the east. From here you have a wonderful view of the granite landscape around Tenaya Lake **(1.5 miles)**. Return to the car the way you came **(2.9 miles)**.

TO THE TRAILHEAD

GPS Coordinates: N37° 49.964' W119° 29.462'
Drive 12.3 miles west of the Tuolumne Meadows Store on CA 120, turning right (north) onto the signposted May Lake Road. Drive 1.8 miles

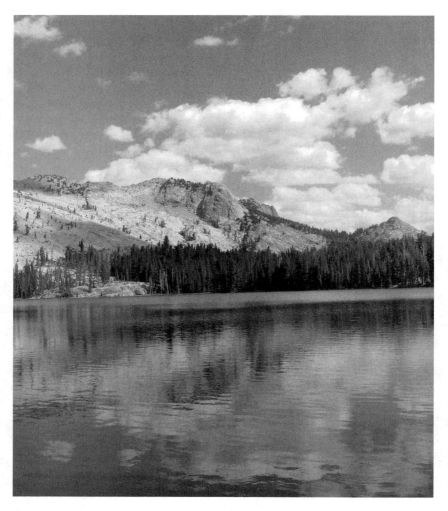

May Lake

north to the parking area at the end of this road. Alternatively, drive 27 miles on CA 120 toward Tuolumne Meadows (east) from Crane Flat before turning left (north) onto May Lake Road and following it 1.8 miles to its end. (Big Oak Flat Road from Yosemite Valley and CA 120 intersect at a T-junction in Crane Flat, located 7.7 miles east of the CA 120 entrance station and 23.7 miles northwest of Yosemite Village.)

26 Mount Hoffmann

Trailhead Location: May Lake Trailhead, 2 miles north of
Tioga Road

Trail Use: Hiking

Distance & Configuration: 5.8-mile out-and-back

Elevation Range: 8,845 feet at the start to 10,850 feet at the summit, with a cumulative elevation change of ±2,040 feet

Facilities: Toilets are available at the trailhead. Drinking water and toilets are available at the May Lake Campground, 1.1 miles into this hike, and at locations in Tuolumne Meadows, the White Wolf High Sierra Camp, and the Crane Flat Store.

Highlights: Unbelievable vista, summit scramble, and May Lake

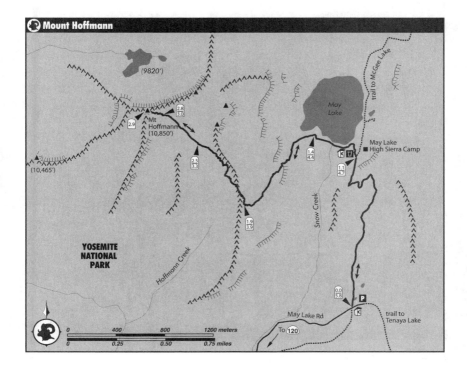

DESCRIPTION

Mount Hoffmann is one of Yosemite's perfectly located gems. It lies at the geographic center of the park, so its 360-degree vista is centered on Yosemite's summits. And it is close enough to Tioga Road—and the trail to May Lake—that it is an easily obtained summit. The final 50 feet to the summit do require a little scrambling, but the slope is not exposed. Take this walk anytime May Lake Road is open, except when a thunderstorm is threatening. Note that the spur road to May Lake often opens several weeks after Tioga Road.

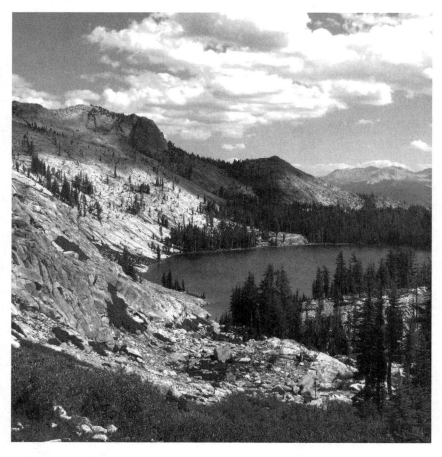

Looking down on May Lake and hemlock groves

THE ROUTE

Departing from the often-buggy parking area, the trail skirts a small tarn and heads north through an open forest. You are crossing slabs covered by just a thin layer of soil—or none at all—as you walk toward May Lake. The trail is initially fairly flat, but the grade increases as you complete two long switchbacks to ascend a dry slope. Beyond, the trail turns east again and enters the predominately mountain hemlock forest that surrounds May Lake's southern shore.

Ahead you spot a junction adjacent to an outhouse and water tap **(1.1 miles from start)**, where straight ahead takes you to the May Lake High Sierra Camp. Instead, take the left-hand fork, which is signposted as the May Lake backpacking camp and is the route to Mount Hoffmann. Several use trails created by hikers meander toward the southern edge of May Lake and then coalesce into a singletrack that skirts the shoreline. The deep-blue waters look very enticing, but note that to protect water quality, swimming is not permitted in May Lake.

Soon after crossing May Lake's outlet stream on logs, the trail passes a knob of bright-white quartzite and turns to the southwest **(1.4 miles)**, diverging from the lake and climbing through a beautiful glade of drooping, pointy-tipped mountain hemlocks. Emerging from tree cover, the trail climbs steeply up an open slope dotted with colorful rock outcrops and pockets of colorful flowers. In places high steps are required to surmount blocks of rock. As you climb, notice that the rock is not granite, for here lies an unusual pocket of the ancient metamorphic rock that overlays the granite. When the trail next levels, you pass a lovely, colorful, and often marshy meadow. Reentering forest cover, you traverse a short distance farther west before turning northwest and resuming a steep rate of ascent **(1.9 miles)**.

The trail leads northwest up an open sandy slope with scattered boulders and stunted whitebark pines. A few tufts of grass and sedges dot the slope, and flowers emerge around the edges of many boulders—their roots seek the greater moisture and warmth beneath the rocks. This stretch is steep and tiring, so take it slow and take care not to slip on sand-covered rocks. The grade lessens when you reach a broad, remarkably vegetated slope beneath Mount Hoffmann's ring of pointy summits **(2.5 miles)**. The high point is the left-most peak, the one topped by antennas, and the trail traipses across the plateau to its base.

Reaching the northern edge of the very steep escarpment **(2.8 miles)**, you begin to climb talus and then often-steep slabs to the summit. The trail now becomes less distinct. Indeed many options exist, all trying to circumvent a majority of boulders and follow stripes of sandy substrate upward. All of course fail to find an idealized route, and you will repeatedly step up onto, over, and down between granite blocks. Fifty feet below the summit, the incline again increases and you are now ascending fractured granite slab. Hands are essential on this section, and parents will likely wish to stand just beneath their children. But don't worry—neither the children nor the adults will have any difficulty ascending.

Within minutes you are standing on the panoramic summit (**2.9 miles**). This summit is aptly named, as Charles Hoffmann, the eponymous cartographer and the first to widely map the Sierra, enjoyed and mapped from this vantage point. Mount Hoffmann is the near-geographic center of Yosemite and is located a considerable distance from taller peaks, providing a view that encompasses most of Yosemite. Half Dome is readily visible to the south, the domes around Tuolumne Meadows can be seen to the east, and the tall peaks along the Sierra Crest form a near semicircle from north to southeast. After a long break, retrace your route to the car (**5.8 miles**).

TO THE TRAILHEAD

GPS Coordinates: N37° 49.964' W119° 29.462'

Drive 12.3 miles west of the Tuolumne Meadows Store on CA 120, turning right (north) onto the signposted May Lake Road. Drive 1.8 miles north to the parking area at the end of this road. Alternatively, drive 27 miles on CA 120 toward Tuolumne Meadows (east) from Crane Flat before turning left (north) onto May Lake Road and following it 1.8 miles to its end. (Big Oak Flat Road from Yosemite Valley and CA 120 intersect at a T-junction in Crane Flat, located 7.7 miles east of the CA 120 entrance station and 23.7 miles northwest of Yosemite Village.)

27 Olmsted Point

Trailhead Location: Tioga Road, east of the May Lake junction and west of Tenaya Lake

Trail Use: Hiking

Distance & Configuration: 0.5-mile out-and-back

Elevation Range: 8,420 feet at the start, with a cumulative elevation change of ±100 feet

Facilities: The closest toilets are at the Sunrise Lake Trailhead at the south end of Tenaya Lake. Water faucets are located at the Tuolumne Meadows Visitor Center and Store, the White Wolf High Sierra Camp, and the Crane Flat Store.

Highlights: Glacier-sculpted granite slabs and Half Dome's and Clouds Rest's steep faces

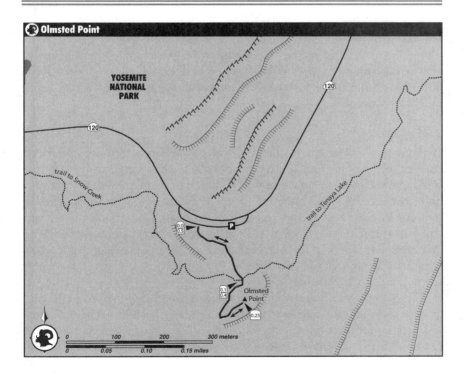

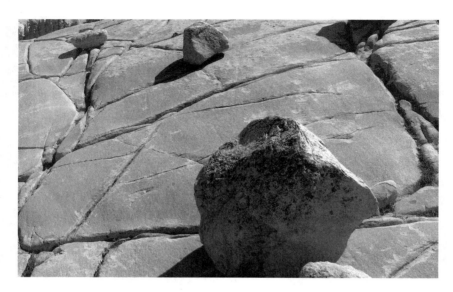

Slabs near Olmsted Point

DESCRIPTION

This short walk takes you beyond the many people enjoying the parking lot view to an even more spectacular overlook of Tenaya Canyon, Clouds Rest, and Half Dome. You can stare at the expansive granite slabs while sitting on a slab yourself.

THE ROUTE

A large sign marks where the trail leads away from the Olmsted Point parking lot; the not-immediately obvious staircase descends from about the middle of the parking area. The trail, at first paved and then dirt, is flanked on either side by small outcrops from which emerge colorful bunches of mountain pride penstemons. You quickly reach an X-junction and continue straight ahead to the lookout **(0.1 mile from start)**. Continue straight, climbing slightly out of the trees and then left onto granite slabs **(0.2 mile)**. Climb to the top of the little dome, Olmsted Point, for the most wide-ranging views **(0.25 mile)**.

The vista is wonderfully characteristic of Yosemite's middle elevations: granite slabs in all directions, advertising many geologic stories. Everywhere is smooth, rounded rock, much of which was once covered with ice. On the far side of Tenaya Canyon is the steep northern face of Half Dome, its approximate shape dictated by fractures in the rock. Clouds Rest is a particular favorite of mine, decorated with steep, undulating avalanche chutes. To the northeast are Tenaya Lake and the steep-faced Mount Conness in the distance. Smaller cracks, allowing soil to collect and trees to grow in an otherwise stark landscape, are visible near you. Look at the junipers and lodgepole pines nearby and on surrounding ridges and notice how they are growing in lines. Also note the scattered boulders, glacial erratics, dropped by the retreating glacier. When you are finished admiring the view, retrace your steps to the car **(0.5 mile)**.

TO THE TRAILHEAD

GPS Coordinates: N37° 48.646' W119° 29.098'

Drive 10 miles west of the Tuolumne Meadows Store on CA 120, turning left (south) into a large parking lot after you climb above Tenaya Lake and then begin a sharp right turn. Alternatively, drive 29.3 miles toward Tuolumne Meadows (east) from Crane Flat. (Big Oak Flat Road from Yosemite Valley and CA 120 intersect at a T-junction in Crane Flat, located 7.7 miles east of the CA 120 entrance station and 23.7 miles northwest of Yosemite Village.)

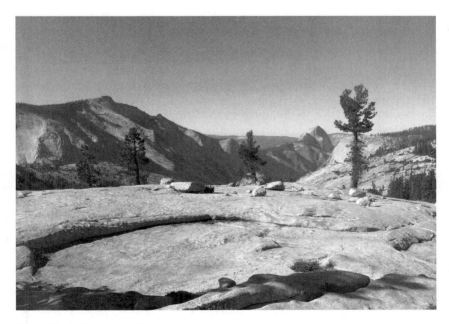

Vista of Clouds Rest and Half Dome

28 Tenaya Lake

Trailhead Location: Tioga Road, at the northern end of Tenaya Lake

Trail Use: Hiking

Distance & Configuration: 2.9-mile loop

Elevation Range: 8,160 feet at the start, with a cumulative elevation change of ±40 feet

Facilities: Toilets are available in the parking area, while the closest water taps are at the Tuolumne Meadows Visitor Center.

Highlights: Granite slab views, sandy beaches, and a beautiful lake

DESCRIPTION

Tenaya Lake is a favorite destination for many recurrent visitors, and this walk lets you enjoy all the lake's best attributes: its sandy beaches, its deep-blue waters, and beautiful views of nearby peaks and domes. Encircling Tenaya Lake is a wonderful walk with young children. The trail is nearly flat, and you can stop just about anywhere for a dip in the remarkably warm water. Unless you are willing to wade the Tenaya Lake outlet, it is best to wait until July to take this walk.

THE ROUTE

From the parking lot to the north of the lake, follow the designated trail to the broad, sandy northern beach. On a windy day, this is a cold location, for the walls to either side of the lake funnel the breezes straight across Tenaya Lake. From this beach, head southeast, away from CA 120. About two-thirds of the way along the beach, you reach a large, deep inlet stream, Tenaya Creek. Head just 50 feet inland to large logs that you can easily balance across. Continue walking along the sandy shore to the end of the beach and then cut through the open lodgepole pine forest for about 75 feet before intersecting the trail along the southeastern shore. This is actually a little-used trail that parallels Tioga Road all the way from Tuolumne Meadows to Tenaya Lake, and you will follow it around the lake's southeastern shore **(0.3 mile from start)**.

Turn southwest (right) onto the trail and trace it through a hemlock and lodgepole pine forest. Your route is slightly set back from the water's

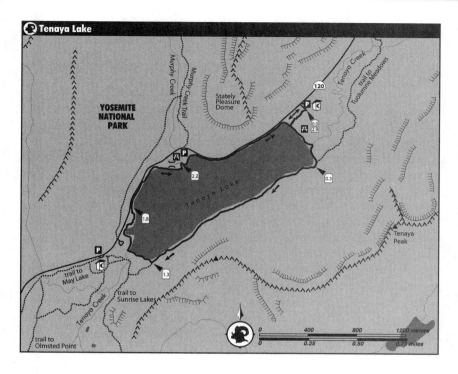

edge, so in places you have filtered views northwest across Tenaya Lake and elsewhere enjoy a sheltered forest walk. This is the least swimmer-friendly side of Tenaya Lake, but if you wish to picnic along its shores, keep your eyes open for one of several shallow, sandy alcoves. The vegetation continues fairly unchanged along most of the southeastern length of the lake, but the forest begins to thin and the views open as you approach the southwestern shore.

Where the water ends **(1.3 miles)**, leave the trail and continue across sand and through small lodgepole pines along the lakeshore. (If you miss the end of the lake and reach a signed junction for Sunrise Lakes, you have gone 0.1 mile too far—backtrack to the end of the lake.) The eastern end of the southwestern shore is another fantastic break location, with few people and exquisite views to the northeast, including Pywiack Dome, the steep dome just to the northeast of the lake, and Stately Pleasure Dome on the northwest side of CA 120. The steep-topped Mount Conness becomes visible as you approach the west corner of the lake. This is the buggiest side of Tenaya Lake, for to the south is a large marshy area along Tenaya Creek's banks. In September a handful of blueberries often wait to be picked from knee-high bushes—keep your eyes open. During early season Tenaya Creek presents a challenge: a notably deep crossing where it connects to Tenaya Lake. If you are visiting in June, expect to get your feet wet, while by mid-summer the outlet runs dry.

Your route now follows use trails created by other hikers as you continue your clockwise walk along the shores. In places you walk on beautiful polished granite slabs, elsewhere along a faint trail through dry grass and sedge meadows. Your path winds closer to and then farther from the water, but the shoreline is never more than 100 feet from you. If you see an enticing spot to stop, the water's edge is nearly always accessible. On a windy day, the southwestern half of the lake tends to be much warmer and the water more inviting than the often windy northeastern beach. About a third of the way around the lake, the shore becomes cumbersome to follow, and you briefly walk close to the edge of the highway **(1.8 miles)** before returning to the lakeshore and passing more busy beaches.

Where Murphy Creek enters the lake, you need to retreat slightly from the lakeshore to cross the fairly narrow, but quite deep, inlet on a log **(2.2 miles)**. Passing a small picnic area, you now find yourself on a sidewalk at the edge of CA 120, your route for the last stretch to the car. Do not let the nearby traffic detract from the advantage of this location, for here no trees block your view of the steep granite slabs to your left (northwest), the popular climbing routes up Stately Pleasure Dome. You can almost always spot climbers ascending the faces and cracks rising above the highway. Turning to your right, notice the stumps emerging from Tenaya Lake's water, remnants of a time when the lake dried up during a severe drought. A short distance along the road takes you back to the northeastern edge of the lake, and you can turn left onto the trail that leads to your car **(2.9 miles)**.

TO THE TRAILHEAD

GPS Coordinates: N37° 50.204' W119° 27.137'

Drive 7.1 miles west of the Tuolumne Meadows Store on CA 120, turning left (east) into a large parking lot shortly before you reach the northeastern shore of Tenaya Lake. The parking lot is not visible from the road and is easy to miss; as you descend a long straightaway with views of granite walls on either side, note the yellow junction sign indicating the parking area entrance. Alternatively, drive 32.2 miles toward Tuolumne Meadows (east) from Crane Flat. The parking area is 0.1 mile beyond the northeastern shore of Tenaya Lake. (Big Oak Flat Road from Yosemite Valley and CA 120 intersect at a T-junction in Crane Flat, located 7.7 miles east of the CA 120 entrance station and 23.7 miles northwest of Yosemite Village.)

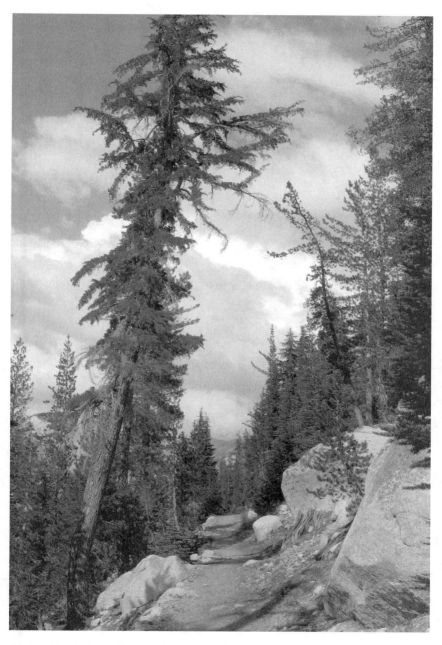

An elegant hemlock along Tenaya Lake's eastern shore

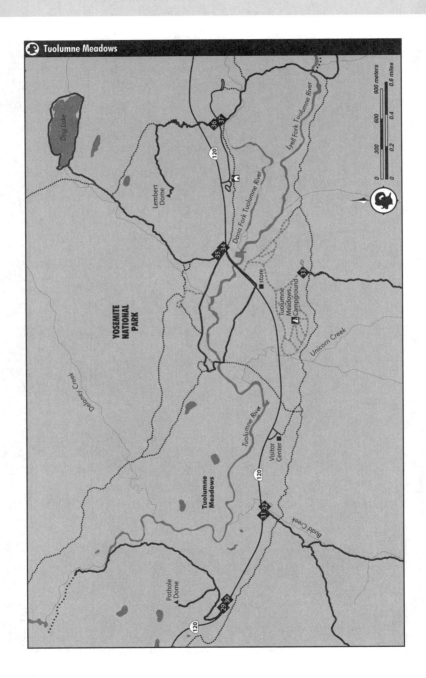

TUOLUMNE MEADOWS

Regional Overview

Tuolumne Meadows is an expansive meadow system flanking the Tuolumne River. Glaciated landforms, including prominent domes (Lembert Dome, Pothole Dome, and Fairview Dome) and steep-summited peaks (Cathedral Peak, Unicorn Peak, and Cockscomb), dominate the view. Elsewhere a thin layer of soil and a conifer forest hide the underlying granite slabs. Above the meadows lie beautiful lakes, glacier-carved granite basins that are filled with water. The lakes to the south of the meadow lie beneath the stunning spires of the Cathedral Range, while the lakes on the north side are generally surrounded by flatter meadows or forest.

Walks in the area fall into three categories: 1) summits or domes, 2) lake destinations, and 3) walks along the Tuolumne River. If time permits, seek out one walk in each class, for they each give a different flavor of Tuolumne Meadows. The summits provide outstanding views of the meadows and peaks, as well as a chance to get up close with glacier-polished granite. Walks to the lakes take you uphill through the forests flanking the meadows, generally with limited views until you reach the stunning bodies of water. The three walks along the Tuolumne River are each different in nature, but all are quite flat.

The selection of hikes includes both shorter walks perfect for an outing with young children and slightly longer adventures better for older kids and adults. In particular, Pothole Dome (Hike 29), Soda Springs and Tuolumne Meadows (Hike 34), and the Tuolumne River (Hike 30) are all suitable for a 4-year-old. Meanwhile children age 6 and up will enjoy the walks to Elizabeth Lake (Hike 33), Lembert Dome (Hike 36), and Dog Lake (Hike 35). Lower Cathedral Lake (Hike 31), Cathedral Peak Shoulder (Hike 32), and Lyell Canyon (Hike 37) are either more difficult or longer and best for children older than age 10.

Tioga Road (CA 120) skirts the southern edge of the meadow, providing easy access to this stunning location from approximately late May–October. During the summer months it is indeed a small town, with amenities including a visitor center, campground, store, grill, post office, gas station, mountaineering store, and the Tuolumne Lodge. Most important for the hiker, a free shuttle bus services stops from Tioga Pass to the east to Olmsted Point to the west. Driving directions are given from the Tuolumne Meadows Store, located on the south side of the road just west of the campground—toward the east end of the meadows. Note that Tioga Road is closed in winter and spring, with exact opening dates determined by snowfall. Moreover, it is usually mid-June or early July before the snowpack is sufficiently melted to complete these walks.

◘ ◘ ◘

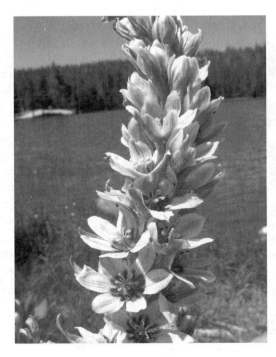

Stalk of corn lily flowers at Dog Lake (see page 160)

29 Pothole Dome

Trailhead Location: West end of Tuolumne Meadows

Trail Use: Hiking

Distance & Configuration: 1.4-mile out-and-back

Elevation Range: 8,605 feet at the start, with 190 feet of ascent/descent

Facilities: No amenities are at this trailhead. Water and restrooms are available at the visitor center, 1.2 miles east along CA 120.

Highlights: Polished granite slabs and expansive Tuolumne Meadows vistas

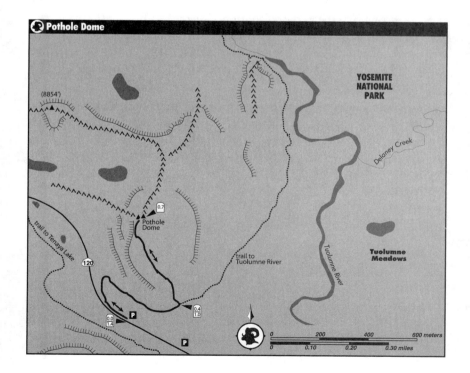

DESCRIPTION

The walk up Pothole Dome is a wonderful family excursion. Even quite young children happily run up the slabs to the top of Pothole Dome, and adults can repeatedly stop and enjoy the ever-more inclusive view of Tuolumne Meadows and the surrounding mountains. Large swaths of rock are still beautifully polished from past glaciers. Feel them with your hands, but walk around them to avoid slipping.

THE ROUTE

From the parking lot, you will be staring north across a narrow tongue of Tuolumne Meadows. At the far side you see a trail and, beyond, the granite slabs of Pothole Dome. Signs and a small fence indicate that the meadow is a restoration area and point you left (west) around the lobe of meadow. In early summer you will not be tempted to ignore the request, for the meadow will be very marshy. But please, also spend the extra 5 minutes later in the season to avoid compacting the soil and damaging the vegetation.

A narrow track leads you first west, then briefly north, and finally east as you encircle the end of Tuolumne Meadows. The southern edge of Pothole Dome now rises steeply to your left. Do not ascend yet; the way up is much gentler. Continue eastward at the edge of the flower-filled meadow. Just after the trail bends left (north), you will notice a faint track

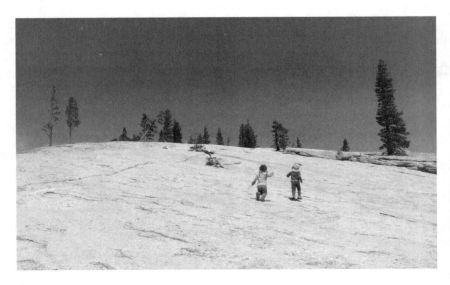

Little legs running up Pothole Dome

to the left, the direction of Pothole Dome. Leave the main trail here—or anywhere for the next 300 feet—walk briefly through lodgepole pine forest, and begin your ascent **(0.4 mile from start)**.

Ahead you see the sloping granite slabs that comprise Pothole Dome. You quickly exit the forest, reach them, and begin climbing. The summit is up and to your right (north). Most people choose to climb straight up to the ridge and then follow the ridge north to the summit, but the only "rule" is that you must stop often to enjoy the expanding view of Tuolumne Meadows. You climb past scattered boulders—glacial erratics, or rocks left behind by retreating glaciers. Indeed, the glaciers once flowed up and over Pothole Dome, giving it its distinctive shape, termed a roche moutonnée. The glacier flowed up the "gentle" slope you are ascending and created a jagged, very steep slope on the downhill side. Glacial polish, the shiny surface that is present on sections of rock, is another indication of past glaciations and formed as grit in the ice was repeatedly pushed over the granite surface, smoothing the rock. Note how slippery the polished sections of rock are and, where possible, select a route that avoids them.

As you approach the ridge, the vista keeps expanding. East of Tuolumne Meadows are two giant reddish-colored peaks that lie along the eastern boundary of Yosemite: Mount Dana and Mount Gibbs. To their north are gray granite peaks, including steep-sided Mount Conness. To the north and west is a landscape of shorter granite slabs and domes interspersed with forest. To the south is the Cathedral Range, a collection of steep summits that rose above the glaciers. Continue north along the mostly flat ridge, climbing one more short stretch to the peak's summit **(0.7 mile)**.

From the summit retrace your steps to the parking lot **(1.4 miles)**. This hike can be combined with Hike 30, the walk to Tuolumne River, by descending Pothole Dome to the trail that skirts the edge of Tuolumne Meadows and continuing north along that trail.

TO THE TRAILHEAD

GPS Coordinates: N37° 52.617' W119° 23.676'

At the far western end of Tuolumne Meadows, 2.1 miles west of the Tuolumne Meadows Store, is a small parking lot on the north side of the road; park in it. Just beyond the parking lot, the road bends right and climbs out of Tuolumne Meadows.

30 Tuolumne River

Trailhead Location: West end of Tuolumne Meadows

Trail Use: Hiking

Distance & Configuration: 3.2-mile out-and-back

Elevation Range: 8,605 feet at the start, with a cumulative elevation change of ±140 feet

Facilities: No amenities are at this trailhead. Water and restrooms are available at the visitor center, 1.2 miles east along CA 120.

Highlights: Late-summer swimming holes and sandy beaches, as well as a slab-lined riverbed

DESCRIPTION

The walk along an unmaintained trail to the Tuolumne River lets you enjoy both the wide meandering river just before it leaves Tuolumne Meadows and the tumbling, bubbling river as it then drops more steeply down granite slabs. In early summer the water is flowing fast and furious, but by late summer the water levels are low, revealing a delightful chain of swimming holes and beaches. Once a near secret, it is now well known among families with children, and by lunchtime the stream banks are lined with picnicking families.

THE ROUTE

Standing outside your car, you look across a narrow lobe of Tuolumne Meadows to a trail skirting Pothole Dome. This is where you are headed, but your route is around the western edge of the meadow to avoid damaging it.

The trail trends first west, paralleling the road, then briefly north, and finally east around the meadow. The southern edge of Pothole Dome rises steeply to your left. Continuing east you walk among scattered lodgepole pine trees at the edge of the meadow. Follow the trail where it bends to the left **(0.4 mile from start)**, tracing the boundary between the meadow (to your right) and lodgepole pine forests (to your left). Although unimproved (in other words, an unofficial use trail), the route is easy to follow. Tuolumne Meadows used to be nearly devoid of trees, but with each decade more lodgepole pines become established, obstructing your view and providing sheltered locations for Tuolumne's large deer population. An observant hiker will spot many animals grazing.

Beyond, the previously distant river converges with the forest boundary **(1.0 mile)**. It is a wide, deep, fairly sluggish meandering course, for Tuolumne Meadows is nearly flat. During spring runoff it swells to its banks or beyond, while by midsummer the waterway is lined by sandbanks, and you might contemplate a cold dip.

Just a few steps later, you leave Tuolumne Meadows and the trail rounds a small buttress; here the river's character instantly changes, for the river gradient steepens. Now a torrent of water rushes over bare granite slabs, pouring into and instantly spilling over deep holes carved in the rock **(1.2 miles)**. Early season safety dictates that you enjoy this scene from the river's bank and keep children under close supervision. However by late July, water levels are low enough that you can safely swim in the deep pools and then bask on the warm slabs or enjoy the sandbanks when you become too cold.

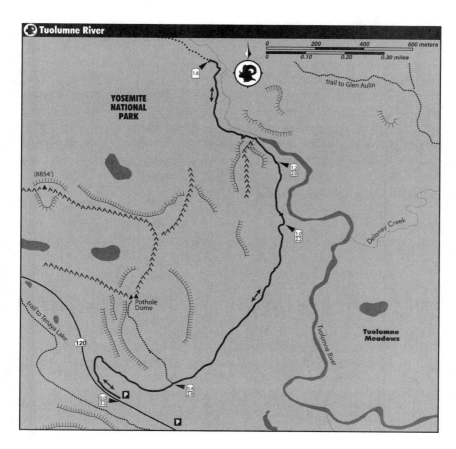

From the point where the stream's gradient increases, continue a short distance to a section of river with many good swimming holes—many options exist **(1.6 miles to lower end of swimming holes)**. Retrace your steps to the car **(3.2 miles)**. If the group has extra energy and time, detour to Pothole Dome (Hike 29) on the return.

TO THE TRAILHEAD

GPS Coordinates: N37° 52.617' W119° 23.676'

At the far western end of Tuolumne Meadows, 2.1 miles west of the Tuolumne Meadows Store, is a small parking lot on the north side of the road; park here. Just beyond the parking lot, the road bends right and climbs out of Tuolumne Meadows.

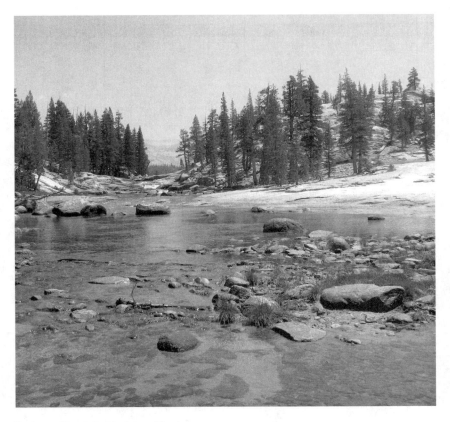

Tuolumne River below Tuolumne Meadows

31 Lower Cathedral Lake

Trailhead Location: West end of Tuolumne Meadows

Trail Use: Hiking

Distance & Configuration: 7.4-mile out-and-back

Elevation Range: 8,570 feet at the start, with a cumulative elevation change of ±1,320 feet

Facilities: Pit toilets are available at this trailhead. Water is available at the Tuolumne Meadows Store and the Tuolumne Meadows Visitor Center, the latter 0.5 mile east along CA 120.

Highlights: Stark granite slabs and peaks, slab-encircled lake, and Cathedral Peak views

DESCRIPTION

One of Yosemite's ultimate destination hikes, this walk takes you through dense forest to reach a spectacular lake—a large, deep glacial-carved (cirque) lake mostly encircled by smooth, polished granite and steep, glacial-carved walls. The walk is pleasant but underwhelming in comparison to the lake and therefore best for children who are old enough to understand a delayed reward.

THE ROUTE

Leaving the trailhead, you head south, directly away from the road. After just 0.1 mile you reach the John Muir Trail at a four-way intersection. The trail to the lower Cathedral Lake, coincident with the John Muir Trail, continues straight ahead, while the left-hand fork is the route that the John Muir Trail follows through Tuolumne Meadows, and the right-hand fork is a track to Tenaya Lake.

The trail climbs steadily up switchbacks through a dense conifer forest before reaching a fairly level shelf **(0.8 mile from start)**. The forest cover is now more open, and the trail repeatedly passes small marshy meadows ringed by stunted, twisted trees, for here flat granite slabs lie not far below the surface, trapping melting snow. In early summer marsh marigolds fill the meadows. Swaths of missing trees indicate where recurring avalanches sweep down from the bare slopes to the left (south). Fairview Dome is visible to the northwest.

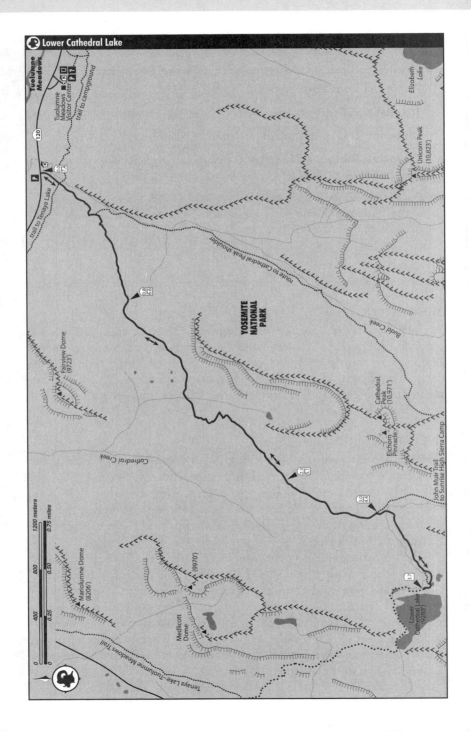

After crossing a small creek—a step-across crossing—the trail resumes its upward trajectory, climbing another 440 feet before leveling off on a dry, sandy flat with scattered tree cover **(2.3 miles)**. You continue through this environment and cross a nearly indiscernible pass, the drainage divide between Tuolumne Meadows (the Tuolumne River) and Yosemite Valley (the Merced River). Cathedral Peak, steep granite slabs culminating in a sharp summit, is now visible to your left. Descending gently, you reenter a denser lodgepole pine forest with more ground cover and occasional open boggy sections.

A short distance later you reach a T-junction. The John Muir Trail continues straight ahead, en route to Yosemite Valley, while you take the right-hand fork to reach the lower Cathedral Lake **(3.0 miles)**. Note that the upper Cathedral Lake is another 0.6 mile along the John Muir Trail. It is another lovely lake but not quite as exquisite as your destination.

The spur trail to the lower Cathedral Lake descends through forest and shortly crosses a stream. A little searching upstream and downstream of the trail crossing will usually reveal a fallen log that you can balance across, but otherwise this is a wet-shoe crossing when water levels are high. Soon the trail emerges from dense forest cover—first next to the banks of the now-meandering stream and after a few more steps you are at the edge of an expansive and often-saturated meadow rimmed by straggly lodgepole pines. The lake is just beyond the meadow but still out of view.

In June and sometimes July this meadow is a shallow lake, for, once again, granite slabs lay not far beneath the surface and the snowmelt pools. The official trail makes a beeline through this marshy mess, crossing the stream twice en route, both times a deep wade. Many people are discouraged by this view and picnic at the forest's edge. Others are rightfully concerned by the potential damage from human feet and search for a less marshy option, resulting in many use tracks in the meadow. A better option is to skirt the southern edge of the meadow; here you will find less soggy soil, can walk mostly on rock, inflict less damage, and stay on the south side of the inlet creek. If you take this detour, make sure that you find a truly dry patch of meadow or slabs to walk on; don't just create a new track through a different stretch of wet meadow. Once the meadow is dry, follow the designated trail due west.

A short jaunt brings you to slabs on the far side of the meadow, and just beyond you see the lakeshore at the base of the steeply sloping slabs **(3.7 miles)**. Small sandy flats among the slabs are beautiful locations for lunch, for you are perched above the lake with views of the water and the surrounding granite walls. Tresidder Peak is the steep mountain overhanging the south side of the lake, while Cathedral Peak rises sharply to the east.

These slabs are not a good location from which to access the water. If your goal is wading or swimming, you will need to walk around to the north side of the lake. To do this, follow the slabs north, back toward the stream. If you stay near the boundary of the meadow and slab, you will reach the creek at a location where its course is wide and shallow and a line of rocks makes it possible to hop across. Beyond the crossing, you pick up a faint trail and follow it through the lodgepole pine forest until you see the lakeshore to your left (south). The side trip to access water is not included in the total trip mileage. Return the way you came **(7.4 miles)**.

TO THE TRAILHEAD

GPS Coordinates: N37° 52.396' W119° 22.967'

The trailhead is toward the western end of Tuolumne Meadows, 1.4 miles west of the Tuolumne Meadows Store. It is on the south side of the road and marked by a row of bear boxes. There is no parking lot, so join the large number of cars parked along the shoulder on both sides of the road. The trail begins just behind the bear boxes.

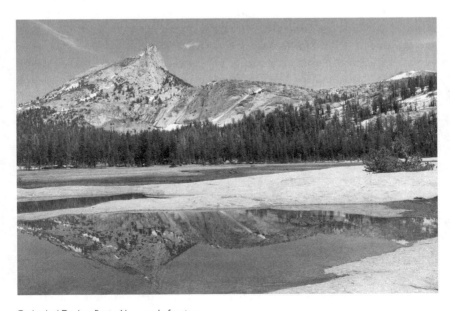

Cathedral Peak reflected in a pool of water

32 Cathedral Peak Shoulder

Trailhead Location: West end of Tuolumne Meadows

Trail Use: Hiking

Distance & Configuration: 5.4-mile out-and-back

Elevation Range: 8,570 feet at the start to 10,120 feet at the summit, with a cumulative elevation change of ±1,600 feet

Facilities: Pit toilets and bear boxes are available at this trailhead. Water is available at the Tuolumne Meadows Store and Tuolumne Meadows Visitor Center, the latter 0.5 mile east along CA 120.

Highlights: Granite spires, granite slabs, and granite walls

DESCRIPTION

Cathedral Peak, a steep horn rising to the south of the meadow, is one of the icons of Tuolumne Meadows. A well-worn climber's trail to the base of the peak allows hikers to ascend to the remarkably flat saddle just south of Cathedral Peak and stare at granite peaks in all directions. This pass is one of my favorite perches in the Cathedral Range.

THE ROUTE

From the Cathedral Lakes parking area, head south through a sandy patch (the old parking lot) and pick up the trail heading south. After 0.1 mile you cross the trail that parallels the south side of Tuolumne Meadows and continue straight ahead on the John Muir Trail toward the Cathedral Lakes. The trail climbs persistently through a dry forest. After ascending about 200 feet, it bends distinctly to the right and then switchbacks back to the left. Now keep your eyes open, for before the trail next bends right, you will depart left onto the unlabeled and unofficial Cathedral Peak climber's trail **(0.4 mile from start)**. A large log intentionally obscures the start of the trail, but just on the back side of the log is a large cairn indicating that you have found the correct location. Do not take this unwelcoming start as an indication of a hard-to-follow trail, for in summer approximately 30 climbers ascend this route each day, and the trail is well etched into the forest floor.

Traversing southeast, you now head toward the west bank of Budd Creek, skirting just above it on the narrow, winding trail. This stretch

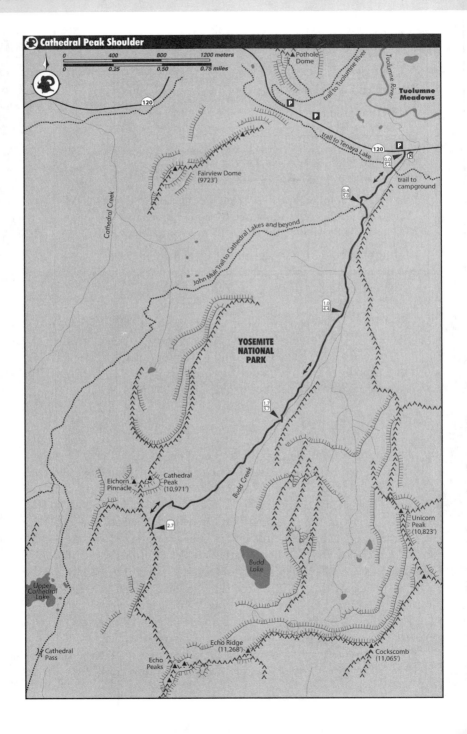

Cathedral Peak Shoulder

0   400   800   1200 meters
0   0.25   0.50   0.75 miles

Pothole Dome

trail to Tuolumne River

Tuolumne River

Tuolumne Meadows

120

trail to Tenaya Lake   120

0.0
5.4

trail to campground

0.4
5.0

Fairview Dome (9723')

John Muir Trail to Cathedral Lakes and beyond

Cathedral Creek

1.0
4.4

YOSEMITE NATIONAL PARK

1.7
3.7

Eichorn Pinnacle   Cathedral Peak (10,971')

Budd Creek

2.7

Unicorn Peak (10,823')

Upper Cathedral Lake

Budd Lake

Cathedral Pass

Echo Ridge (11,268')

Echo Peaks

Cockscomb (11,065')

displays the benefits of a built trail, for here there are endless small undulations and logs to climb across. Luckily, you soon step across a small side creek and diverge from the stream banks, crossing through a lodgepole pine flat and then emerging on open slabs **(1.0 mile)**. The trail crosses up and right across the slabs into a narrow gully on the slabs' right side. The trail of course disappears on the slabs, but simply continue straight up, jogging right where cairns indicate a turn. On the far side of the slabs, the trail is again obvious as it ascends in slots past short, steep outcrops. Do not continue beyond the slabs until you locate the continuation of the trail.

Now on a shallow crest again, you are suddenly treated to outstanding views of Unicorn Peak (to the east) and Cockscomb (to the southeast), with an amazing expanse of steep slab in the foreground. Diverging from Unicorn Peak, the trail descends once again to the banks of Budd Creek **(1.7 miles)**. A use trail to Budd Lake crosses the creek here and ascends the east (left) bank, while you continue climbing on the right-hand (west)

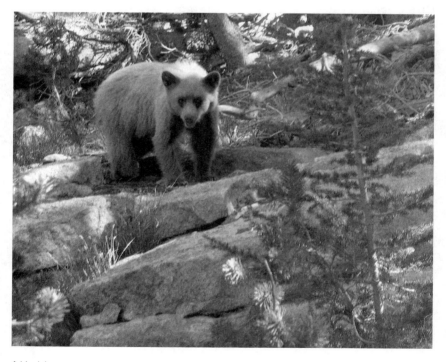

A black bear

side. Ascending back into dry, open lodgepole pine forest, Cathedral Peak is now to your right, a single steep spire emerging above the glistening granite slabs. After a section of denser forest, the trail turns to the right and begins climbing quite steeply, ascending the final slope to the base of Cathedral Peak. Climb up until you are at the same elevation as the shallow saddle in front and to the left of you, and then leave the climber's trail and walk across open sandy slopes and slabs to the pass **(2.7 miles)**.

Sit on a boulder and enjoy the view! The Echo Peaks are the collection of spires due south, while Echo Ridge extends out farther east. To the southwest is Tresidder Peak and below are the Cathedral Lakes. To the north are the peaks of northern Yosemite, including steep-faced Mount Conness. This is a wonderful location from which to imagine the glaciers covering the landscape, including where you are sitting, while the surrounding spires emerged above the ice. After an enjoyable break, retrace your steps to the car **(5.4 miles)**.

TO THE TRAILHEAD
GPS Coordinates:
N37° 52.396' W119° 22.967'
Toward the western end of Tuolumne Meadows, 1.4 miles west of the Tuolumne Meadows Store, the trailhead on the south side of the road is marked by a row of bear boxes. There is no parking lot, so join the large number of cars parked along the shoulder on both sides of the road. The trail begins just behind the bear boxes.

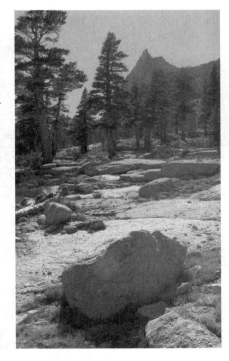

View to Cathedral Peak

33 Elizabeth Lake

Trailhead Location: Back of Tuolumne Meadows Campground

Trail Use: Hiking

Distance & Configuration: 4.2-mile out-and-back

Elevation Range: 8,660 feet at the start to 9,487 feet at the turn-around point, with a cumulative elevation change of ±850 feet

Facilities: A toilet block and water faucet are located at the parking area.

Highlights: Unicorn Peak views, heath-ringed lake, pinecones, and conifer bark

DESCRIPTION

Name aside, Elizabeth Lake has always been a favorite family walk, for it is not too long and not too steep, and it departs directly from the Tuolumne Meadows Campground, eliminating the hassle of first driving (or taking the shuttle bus) to a trailhead if you are camping. You walk through varied and engaging forest, with beautiful pinecones to admire, eventually reaching a picturesque lake set against the striking summit pinnacle of Unicorn Peak.

THE ROUTE

Heading south, you immediately reach an X-junction with the trail that skirts the southern edge of Tuolumne Meadows. Continue straight ahead. The trail to Elizabeth Lake climbs up a not-too-steep slope to the east of Unicorn Creek. There are few switchbacks as you ascend through the mixed conifer forest, with stretches of steeper trail dominated by dense mountain hemlocks and white firs, while flatter bits are open lodgepole pine forest. The understory is composed of crisscrossing downed logs and scattered flowers, especially lupines and wandering daisies. Only a small step-across creek interrupts your path **(0.5 mile from start)**.

After crossing a second creek on a pair of downed logs **(1.1 miles)**, you climb onto a shallow ridge with filtered views to the north. The grade now lessens, as you first walk along an old lateral moraine—the rock and silt deposits left along the edge of a retreating glacier—and then into a flat stretch of lodgepole pine forest. Here lies a dense understory of dwarf

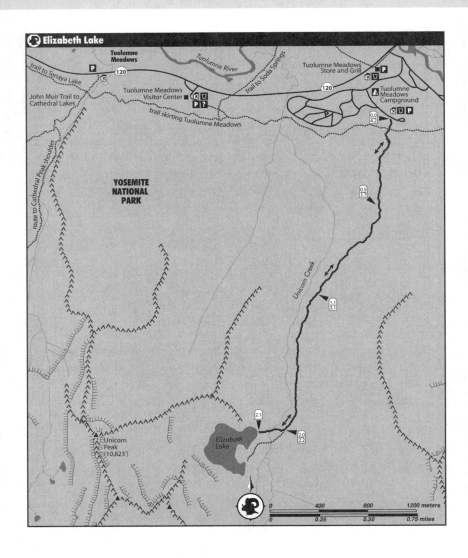

bilberry, a blueberry relative that unfortunately rarely produces fruit. The lodgepole pines tell a story of trying winters, for the young trees are bent and contorted from the weight of the winter snowpack. As they grow taller, the trees are finally able to emerge above the snow and slowly become straighter with age.

Continuing along, Unicorn Peak becomes ever more prominent to the right, and shortly you reach a T-junction where you turn right to the lakeshore **(2.0 miles)**. The left-hand fork is shown as the trail on most maps, and it is indeed a beautiful route. However, it leads to a crossing of Unicorn Creek that is deep and a bit wide for a jump, meaning that it cannot easily be completed with dry feet. In contrast, turning right leads to a crossing on rocks and just beyond the shores of Elizabeth Lake **(2.1 miles)**. Relax at the first lakeside location you reach, or continue around the lake for different views, (cold) swimming options, or shade. The best views of Unicorn Peak are from the northeastern shores, near the outlet stream. Return to the campground the way you came **(4.2 miles)**, or first take a little detour south to enjoy beautiful meadows farther along Unicorn Creek.

TO THE TRAILHEAD
GPS Coordinates: N37° 52.234' W119° 21.350'
A day-use trailhead for Elizabeth Lake is located inside the Tuolumne Meadows Campground. From the Tuolumne Meadows Store, turn left (east) onto CA 120. Continue for just 0.1 mile before turning right into the campground. Continue straight ahead for 0.1 mile to the entrance kiosk, let the attendant know your destination, and then take a right-hand turn in the directions of loops B–G. After an additional 0.2 mile take a prominent left-hand turn toward the group sites and B sites 38–49. Continue straight, past the turnoff from the group sites, and after another 0.2 mile you will come to a parking area. The trail departs to the northwest. If you reach the horse camp, you have gone too far.

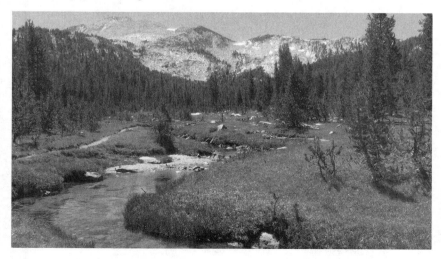

Meadow corridor near Elizabeth Lake

34 Soda Springs and Tuolumne Meadows

Trailhead Location: Lembert Dome parking lot

Trail Use: Hiking

Distance & Configuration: 1.9-mile loop or 1.8-mile out-and-back

Elevation Range: 8,590 feet at the start, with a cumulative elevation change of ±30 feet

Facilities: Toilets are at the initial parking lot, but no water is available here. Fill your water bottles at the Tuolumne Meadows Store, backcountry office, or campground.

Highlights: Soda Springs, Parsons Lodge, meadow walking, and a ring of mountains

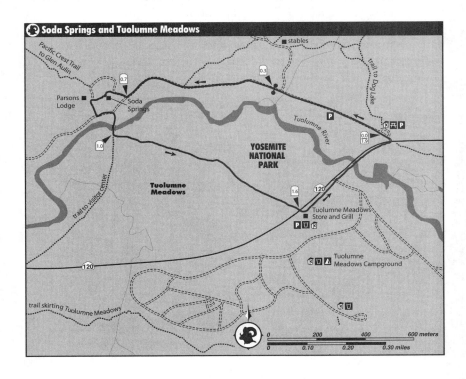

DESCRIPTION

Most trailheads in the Tuolumne Meadows region begin by *leaving* the meadows. They disappear into the conifer forests that surround the gigantic meadow. If you just want to absorb the beautiful flower-filled meadow and look up at the surrounding peaks, take this walk. You will also visit the intriguing Soda Springs and the historic Parsons Lodge. During June the second half of this loop will be too muddy to complete, so make it an out-and-back walk to Parsons Lodge.

THE ROUTE

Leaving the parking lot, head northwest on the straight dirt road; it is usually lined with cars because it is used as the overflow from the Lembert Dome parking lot. When you come to a locked gate **(0.3 mile from start)**, slip around it and continue your walk through an open lodgepole pine forest. Shortly you leave tree cover and enter the meadow. Information placards, providing information on glaciers, meadow wildlife, and more, line the trail. Several spectacular granite summits are visible: Unicorn and Cathedral peaks are the two pinnacle-topped mountains to the southwest, while Fairview Dome is

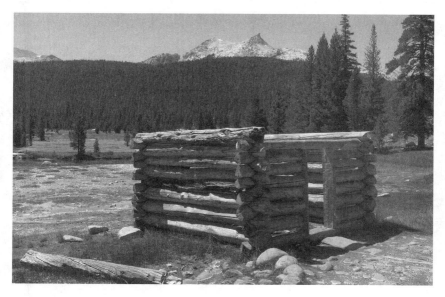

Cabin built to protect the Soda Springs

the large, steep-sided dome to the right of Cathedral Peak. Pothole Dome (Hike 29), an easy Tuolumne destination, is visible to the west.

At a Y-junction, a spur trail to the right is signposted as the route to Glen Aulin and the Pacific Crest Trail, while the dirt road you have been following bends to the left **(0.7 mile)**. Leave the road and take the right-hand fork up a short slope. Within 2 minutes you reach a second junction: right is again marked as the route to Glen Aulin, while the left branch takes you to Soda Springs and Parsons Lodge across a meadow. Head left, walking slowly along the stone-tiled trail toward a small wooden structure. Walk slowly because the first attractions are small springs bubbling out of the soil. Many more are located inside the log enclosure, built in 1885 to protect them from the hooves of the sheep that once grazed here. Early visitors to Tuolumne Meadows would sample this pure water, the bubbles likely the result of volcanic activity deep underground.

Beyond the Soda Springs you reach Parsons Lodge, built in 1915 as a meeting place for the Sierra Club. Today it houses a wonderful collection of historical information on Tuolumne Meadows and the Sierra Club; it is well worth your time to explore this "museum." Afterward, head from the cabin's front door down to the Tuolumne River, meeting up with the dirt road you had previously been following, briefly heading east (left) and then crossing a beautiful bridge **(1.0 mile)**. Look over the railing at the rounded cobbles on the river bottom and west across Tuolumne Meadows.

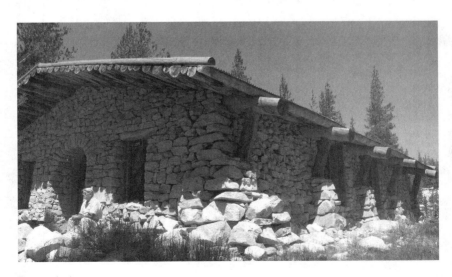

Parsons Lodge

Once across the bridge, the main trail continues straight across the meadow, eventually crossing CA 120 near the Tuolumne Meadows Visitor Center. However, just beyond the bridge, you diverge to the left, crossing the meadow on an unofficial use trail that parallels the Tuolumne River toward the Tuolumne Meadows Store. If this use trail is boggy or muddy, such as in early summer, please turn around at this point and return the way you came to avoid damaging the meadow; wet soil compacts under your feet, making it less hospitable to plant roots. From the bridge, turn and face Parsons Lodge; now turn right (east) onto the dirt road. You will shortly reconnect with your route from earlier and retrace your steps to the car. During most of the summer and fall, however, you can continue the loop, allowing you to immerse yourself in Tuolumne's expansive meadows.

As you head east on the use trail, Lembert Dome rises steeply in front of you. Stop from time to time and turn around to enjoy the steep shapes of Unicorn Peak to the east and Cathedral Peak to the west. Over 2 short months, the meadow's color shifts from an intense yellow-green in spring to a vibrant green midsummer and a burnt yellow in fall. Indeed, the alpine summer is so short that different species bloom each week, but there are always a few flowers to enjoy. The track crosses a small, usually dry, tributary stream and continues across more flower-filled meadows, eventually reaching CA 120 across the street from the Tuolumne Meadows Store **(1.6 miles)**.

Cross the street, for the north side of the street does not have a good pedestrian option. Walk along the edge of the road, past the campground entrance, and across the bridge over the Tuolumne River. Continue along the edge of a large meadow until you see the Lembert Dome parking area on the left (north) side of the street. Cross the street and find your car **(1.9 miles)**.

TO THE TRAILHEAD

GPS Coordinates: N37° 52.639' W119° 21.206'
From the Tuolumne Meadows Store, turn left (east) onto CA 120. Continue for 0.3 mile, past the campground, across a bridge, and immediately to a junction. Turn left onto the spur road. To your right is the small Lembert Dome parking area. If you find a parking spot, stop here. Otherwise loop through the parking area, turn right (northwest), and continue along the dirt road. For the next 0.3 mile (until you reach a locked gate), you may park along the edge of the dirt road. As this is also part of your walking route, it does not matter exactly where you park.

35 Dog Lake

Trailhead Location: Lembert Dome parking lot

Trail Use: Hiking

Distance & Configuration: 2.4- to 3.6-mile out-and-back

Elevation Range: 8,590 feet at the start, with 580 feet of ascent/descent

Facilities: Toilets are at the initial parking lot, but no water is available here. Fill your water bottles at the Tuolumne Meadows Store, backcountry office, or campground.

Highlights: Colorful lakeside meadows, sandy swimming beaches, and secretive mountain views

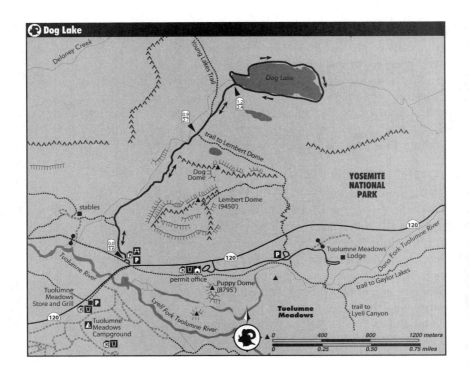

DESCRIPTION

Dog Lake is often selected as a destination simply because it is one of Tuolumne Meadows's shorter walks—an unfair depiction of a beautiful forest-ringed lake with some of the region's best swimming beaches. The water is warm, or at least warmer than most mountain lakes, and the lakeside meadows are brightly colored with flowers. This walk is accessible as soon as the snow has melted, but it's best after mid-July when mosquitoes are less abundant.

THE ROUTE

Leaving the parking area, follow the trail past the restrooms and into a small patch of lodgepole pine forest before crossing a blindingly bright stretch of polished granite slabs extending off Lembert Dome. You will find excellent views of Tuolumne Meadows from this location. Passing two left-bearing junctions to the Tuolumne Meadows Stables, you stay straight ahead each time. The trail now turns to the right and begins to climb more steeply, following the side of the Dog Lake outlet stream. In places you are near the verdant and flower-lined creek banks and elsewhere on a quite steep, dry slope of lodgepole pines. As you ascend, you cross a small side creek—a step across most of the time and on downed logs if water levels are quite high. Shortly after, you diverge for good from the creek and reach a T-junction; continue straight ahead to Dog Lake (and Young Lakes), while right takes you around the back of Lembert Dome **(0.9 mile from start)**.

Climbing more gently now, you reach a Y-junction, where you head right toward Dog Lake, while the left branch leads to the more distant Young Lakes. It is an open landscape, dotted with lodgepole pines and sprinkled with granite boulders. Heading over a small, sandy ridge, you descend briefly and reach the shores of Dog Lake **(1.2 miles)**. Walking to the lakeshore, you look across at the large red masses of Mount Dana and Mount Gibbs, along Yosemite's eastern boundary. You may choose to stop here, but assuming the mosquitoes are not too vicious, I recommend that you traipse around the lake. An unofficial use trail exists most of the way, and the best swimming beaches are scattered along the north shore.

Assuming that you continue, proceed in a clockwise direction, following the trail that heads left. This loop is a quiet, relaxing walk. You begin by stepping across the outlet stream and then skirting briefly away from the lakeshore to avoid a bit of marshy meadow. Other parties may be in search of similarly private sandy beaches, but there are plenty of shallow bays to go around—just pick one along the northern shore, for the southern side is reedy and forested. Along Dog Lake's northern shore, the trail is mostly in the meadow, occasionally passing stately lodgepole pines overlooking the lake. When you reach the eastern end of Dog Lake, you will discover that it is quite marshy; if you are visiting in early season, walk a distance in from the lake to avoid damaging the sensitive meadow vegetation and compacting the wet soils. This is of course also a wonderfully colorful area with light purple shooting stars, burgundy Lemmon's paintbrushes, and lilac alpine asters all vying for your attention. Stepping across the narrow outlet, you reach the southern side of the lake and enter forest cover. It is a remarkable change from the previously sunny shores. Now the banks are lined with shade-dwelling shrubs and flowers, and the forest extends nearly to the lake's banks.

Returning to Dog Lake's outlet **(2.4 miles)**, you pick up the trail you ascended earlier and retrace your steps to the Lembert Dome parking area **(3.6 miles)**.

TO THE TRAILHEAD
GPS Coordinates: N37° 52.639' W119° 21.206'
From the Tuolumne Meadows Store, turn left (east) onto CA 120. Continue for 0.3 mile, past the campground, across a bridge, and immediately to a junction. Turn left onto the spur road. On your right is the small Lembert Dome parking area. If you find a parking spot, stop here. Otherwise loop through the parking area and turn right (northwest) back onto the spur road. For the next 0.3 mile (until you reach a locked gate), you may park along the edge of the dirt road. The trailhead departs from the back of the Lembert Dome parking lot, so pick the first parking spot you see along the spur road.

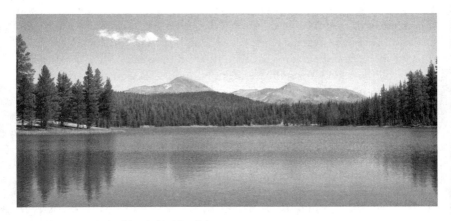

Mount Dana and Mount Gibbs behind Dog Lake

36 Lembert Dome

Trailhead Location: Tuolumne Meadows Lodge Road

Trail Use: Hiking

Distance & Configuration: 2.4-mile out-and-back

Elevation Range: 8,700 feet at the start to 9,450 feet at the summit, with 750 feet of ascent/descent

Facilities: There are no amenities at this parking area. Fill your water bottles and use the toilet at the Tuolumne Meadows Store, permit office, or campground.

Highlights: 360-degree Tuolumne Meadows views, smooth granite slabs, and a must-visit summit

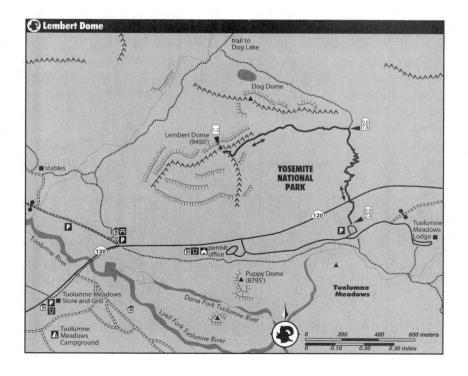

DESCRIPTION

If you have time for just one Tuolumne Meadows walk, it should be an ascent of Lembert Dome (or Pothole Dome, Hike 29, if you are uneasy about scrambling up steep slabs). From the summit you can enjoy the best views of Tuolumne Meadows as you stare out across the expanse of mountain-ringed meadow. Sitting on top, imagine a river of ice flowing up and over your perch, smoothing and polishing the granite you are climbing. Take this walk anytime Tioga Road is open, except when a thunderstorm is threatening.

THE ROUTE

Heading north from the parking lot, the trail ascends a short, steep slope, in part outfitted with granite steps, to reach CA 120. Crossing the road, the trail continues to switchback up a rather steep lodgepole pine–covered slope. Use the abundant downed logs as benches for breathers and find (but don't pick!) a rainbow of flowers as you climb. This slope has a lusher selection of grass tufts and wildflowers than most lodgepole pine forests. The grade lessens as you approach a gentle saddle, and just before reaching the pass, you come to a T-junction **(0.6 mile from start)**. You turn left and head west, while the trail straight ahead leads around the back of Lembert Dome, eventually intersecting the trail to Dog Lake (Hike 35).

You are now on a rougher trail and climb gently through forest and past increasing numbers of slabs, always just to the south (left) of a small ridge. When you emerge on open slabs, you are on a saddle that lies between Lembert Dome (to the southwest) and its shorter, northern summit, nicknamed Dog Dome.

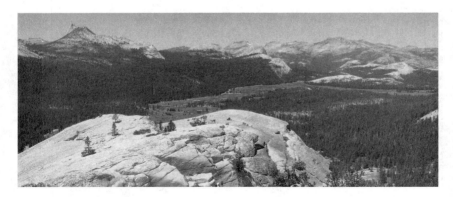

Looking across Tuolumne Meadows from the summit

The trail now ends, but your destination is obvious: the large mass of granite in front of and above you. Turning a little to the left (southwest), you walk first across nearly flat slabs, even dropping a few feet, while noting steepening slabs up the final 60 feet to the summit. Once you are just below the final slope, skirt a little to the south (left) of the ridgeline to bypass the steepest rock. After you have skirted around the first steep bit, you turn right and begin a diagonal ascent to the summit. As you walk up the slabs, keep your soles flat on the rock to maximize friction. Above and to your right a narrow shelf exists in the rock, a good pathway for your feet. You then reach the final 25-foot ascent, most easily climbed via some cracks. The cracks make handholds, making you feel that extra bit secure as you climb from one granite shelf to the next. Children should have no difficulty with the climb, but make sure they don't clown around, as there are steep drop-offs in all directions.

Within a few steps you find yourself at the summit. Stop and enjoy the panoramic view (**1.2 miles**). To the east are red-colored Mount Dana and Mount Gibbs. To the southwest are the twin peaks of Unicorn Peak and the sharp spire of Cathedral Peak. Directly west you stare across Tuolumne Meadows to Mount Hoffmann, Tuolumne Peak, and a never-ending expanse of polished granite. All the rounded domes and undulating granite slabs were once covered with ice, while the sharp-pointed peaks, termed horns, remained above the glacier. Lembert Dome is actually a landform termed a roche moutonnée. The glacier smoothed and polished its upstream (eastern) side, where you have been walking, into a relatively shallow slope, while it plucked rocks from the steep and jagged downstream (western) side.

When you are finished imbibing the view, return the way you came (**2.4 miles**).

TO THE TRAILHEAD
GPS Coordinates: N37° 52.701' W119° 20.339'
From the Tuolumne Meadows Store, turn left (east) onto CA 120. Continue for 0.7 mile, past the campground, across a bridge, and just begin the climb out of Tuolumne Meadows. Very soon you will see a spur road on the right to the Tuolumne Meadows Lodge, Tuolumne Meadows Lodge Road. Turn here, shortly bend to the left, continue for 0.4 mile, and then turn into a large parking area on your left (north). The trail departs from the north end of the parking lot. Alternative parking is available at the permit office parking lot, on the right just after you turned onto Tuolumne Meadows Lodge Road.

37 Lyell Canyon

Trailhead Location: Tuolumne Meadows Lodge Road

Trail Use: Hiking

Distance & Configuration: 1.6- to 7.6-mile out-and-back

Elevation Range: 8,680 feet at the start, with a cumulative elevation change of ±200 feet

Facilities: There are no amenities at this parking area. Fill your water bottles and use the toilet at the Tuolumne Meadows Store, permit office, or campground.

Highlights: Deep, meandering creek; river-smoothed rock; and meadows

DESCRIPTION

Lyell Canyon is one of Yosemite's backcountry treasures that can be enjoyed on a not-too-arduous day hike. There are two particular highlights on this quite flat trek through lodgepole pine forest and across many small meadows. The first is the pair of bridges across the Lyell Fork of the Tuolumne River, for beneath the bridges is some exquisite water-carved rock. The second is the last mile of this walk, when you are in Lyell Canyon proper, a 6-mile-long classically U-shaped glacial canyon, through which flows the deep and meandering Lyell Fork of the Tuolumne River.

THE ROUTE

Departing from the car, you cross the road and find a trailhead marked by one of Yosemite's ubiquitous metal trail markers. You begin your walk paralleling the mostly unseen Dana Fork of the Tuolumne River on a flat trail through lodgepole pine forest. Soon you reach a junction **(0.2 mile from start)**, where left (north) takes you to the Tuolumne Meadows High Sierra Camp and right (southeast) across a newly refurbished bridge. Head across the bridge and continue walking through a dry forest. At a second junction with a trail to Gaylor Lakes, again head right. The trail undulates slightly, mimicking the topography of the underlying granite slabs, and soon you descend a short stretch of dry, open, slabby landscape and come to a second bridge, this one crossing the Lyell Fork of the Tuolumne River **(0.8 mile)**.

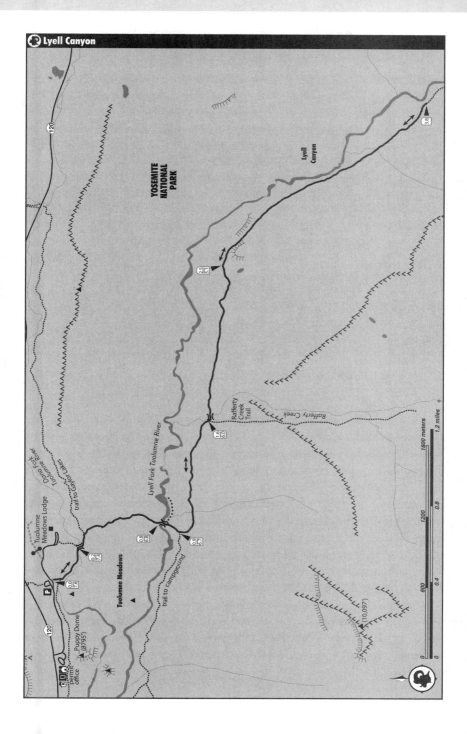

Lyell Canyon

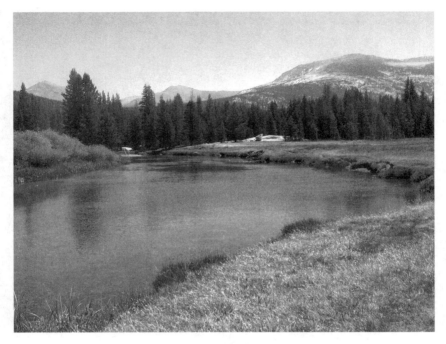

Lyell Fork of the Tuolumne River near the twin bridges

You may be surprised to cross two forks of the Tuolumne River, for a single river flows beneath CA 120 and through the main length of Tuolumne Meadows; these two rivers merge in the broad meadow near the entrance to the Tuolumne Meadows Campground. The Lyell Fork is the larger of the two tributaries, and the bridge crosses it in a spectacular location. The force of runoff has carved exquisite holes and polished "waterslides" in the riverbed and its banks. By late summer water levels are sufficiently low to make swimming and water play safe. Upstream is a long meadow with red-colored Mounts Dana and Gibbs visible in the distance. Many people make this their destination, but I encourage ambitious walkers to continue farther to see the river in a lazier pose.

Beyond the crossing, the trail skirts the meadow and reaches a T-junction **(0.9 mile)**. The right-hand fork is a forested trail that runs the length of Tuolumne Meadows, taking you to the Tuolumne Meadows Campground and Visitor Center. Your route is the left-hand choice, the John Muir Trail, which continues along the meadow and then back into lodgepole pine forest. Much of the trail is in the dry forest, but you also pass open grassy glades densely colored with white yampahs in July and August. Reaching another T-junction, stay straight ahead and cross Rafferty Creek on a wooden bridge **(1.6 miles)**. (The right-hand fork is the Rafferty Creek Trail that climbs to Vogelsang High Sierra Camp.)

The nearly flat trail continues alternating between forest cover and meadow. Stretches of trail near meadows are often muddy in spring and early summer. As you walk, consider the environmental damage caused as each hiker decides to avoid the mud and tramples new bits of meadow, simply creating a new mud wallow. Until August, only take this trail if you are prepared to get slightly muddy shoes and possibly damp feet. You are continuing to parallel the unseen river. It even flows along the far side of some of the meadows you cross, but you cannot actually see it. Slowly the trail begins to bend left, and you pass between two small granite knobs and enter Lyell Canyon **(2.5 miles)**.

Shortly you leave forest cover and find that you are now in a wide glacial canyon. To the east the steep avalanche path–ridden slopes of Mammoth Peak descend to the valley floor, while those to the west are hidden from view. You alternatively walk through the meadow and then detour back into the lodgepole pine forest just to the west, all the while staring up canyon and absorbing the grandeur of the location. You need to continue at least a mile up Lyell Canyon to reach the most wonderful stretch of canyon, where you can enjoy the lazily meandering and often quite deep Lyell Fork of the Tuolumne River and verdant flower-filled meadows extending far beyond the river's banks **(3.8 miles)**. But of course everywhere is perfect for a quiet picnic. Continue until you find a spot that grabs your fancy. Afterward, retrace your steps to the trailhead **(7.6 miles)**.

TO THE TRAILHEAD

GPS Coordinates: N37° 52.663' W119° 20.310'

From the Tuolumne Meadows Store, turn left (east) onto CA 120. Continue for 0.7 mile, past the campground, across a bridge, and just begin the climb out of Tuolumne Meadows. Almost immediately you will see a spur road on the right to the Tuolumne Meadows Lodge, Tuolumne Meadows Lodge Road. Turn here, shortly bend to the left, continue for 0.4 mile, and then turn into a large parking area on your left (north). The trail departs from the south side of Tuolumne Meadows Lodge Road, opposite the parking area. Alternative parking is available at the permit office parking lot, on the right just after you turned onto Tuolumne Meadows Lodge Road.

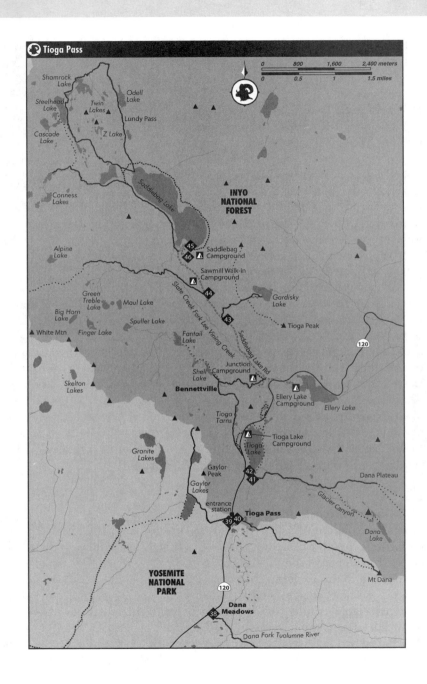

Tioga Pass

TIOGA PASS

Regional Overview

The Tioga Pass region includes the far eastern reaches of Yosemite National Park and onward to Saddlebag Lake, a 10-minute drive east of the park boundary. With trailhead elevations between 9,700 and 10,100 feet, you begin in the subalpine zone where tree cover is becoming sparser, and on most walks you climb into the treeless alpine zone. The rewards on these walks are exquisite alpine lakes, truly expansive mountain views, and simply a feeling of endless space. Jagged alpine summits and ridges decorate the horizon on all the walks described—either steep, smooth granite or jagged, red metamorphic rocks. The Tioga Pass region was the location of a brief mining boom in the 1880s, and relics of this era, including old cabins, tunnels, and mining equipment, still exist in many locations.

While the walks described here all lie close together, each has a remarkably different feel. The lakes and surrounding peaks each have their own personalities. In some locations the lakes dominate the mood (for example, Gaylor Lakes), elsewhere it is the surrounding peaks (for example, Twenty Lakes Basin), and on still other hikes just the feeling of being in the mountains prevails (that is, Mono Pass and Slate Creek). Read the Highlights, which capture the essence of the walks, to decide what attracts you most on a given day.

The ascent of Mount Dana is the most challenging walk described in this book, with a 3,000-foot climb to the 13,057-foot summit, but many of the walks described here are very accessible to children over the age of 5. The two easiest are Bennettville (Hike 42) and Slate Creek (Hike 44), but the walks to Gaylor Lakes (Hike 39, excluding the mines), Conness Lakes (Hike 46), Gardisky Lake (Hike 43), and Twenty Lakes Basin

(Hike 45) also involve less than 1,000 feet of elevation gain. Twenty Lakes Basin receives the greatest traffic in the region, for walks here combine mountain views with lakes and meadows, and a ferry allows hikers to miss the more monotonous miles around Saddlebag Lake. Unfortunately, this ferry is also a bit of a headache, for in summer, even midweek, hikers can wait 2 hours for a spot. Consider taking one of the nearby walks, such as Bennettville (Hike 42), Gardisky Lake (Hike 43), or Slate Creek (Hike 44), that are similarly beautiful and much emptier.

As you embark on a Tioga Pass hike, remember that this is a region of extremes—frigid winter temperatures, strong chilly winds (even in summer), and glaring sun. It is essential to wear hats, sunglasses, and sunscreen and carry a jacket when venturing out at this elevation. Because you are at high elevation, expect to walk more slowly than at sea level, drink plenty of water, and simply take it easy, for there is a lot less oxygen in the air than your body is used to. Tioga Road is usually open late May–October, but due to the large snowpack, the high elevation hiking season rarely begins before early July.

◘ ◘ ◘

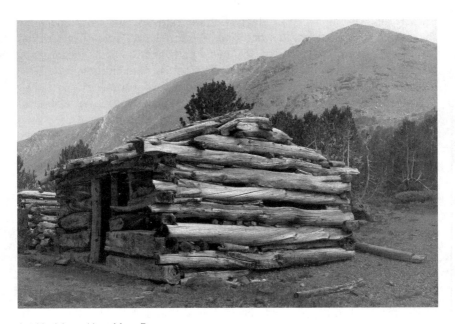

An old mining cabin at Mono Pass

38 Mono Pass

Trailhead Location: Tioga Road east of Tuolumne Meadows

Trail Use: Hiking

Distance & Configuration: 8.0-mile out-and-back

Elevation Range: 9,690 feet at the start, with a cumulative elevation change of ±1,050 feet

Facilities: A pit toilet is at the trailhead, but you must fill water bottles at the Tuolumne Meadows Store or Campground.

Highlights: Old mining cabins, steep walls at the head of Bloody Canyon, and lodgepole pine forests

DESCRIPTION

The hike to Mono Pass is a destination hike. The walk is enjoyable and pleasantly easy, while the subalpine scenery surrounding Mono Pass and the Golden Crown and Ella Bloss mines is simply spectacular. The weathered orange timbers of the mining cabins, the red walls at the head of Bloody Canyon, and the large meadows create a landscape of vibrant colors.

THE ROUTE

Leaving the trailhead (and reading the information placard about the region's mining history), you promptly cross the increasingly treed southern edge of Dana Meadows and cross an unnamed creek and immediately thereafter the Dana Fork of the Tuolumne River **(0.5 mile from start)**. In early summer, these can be challenging crossings with fast-flowing water. The first creek might get your feet wet, and the Dana Fork currently has a log to balance across. By late summer you can easily hop across both creeks on rocks.

The trail bends left (east) and ascends an old moraine. In places you can see the boulders of many different sizes that comprise it. Beyond, the trail bends right, continuing mostly through dense lodgepole pine forest at the base of Mount Gibbs and passing a dilapidated cabin. Your first expansive views come only when you intersect Parker Pass Creek **(1.3 miles)**, which follows a broad meadowed corridor that bends sharply west where you reach it. Continuing under tree cover, you get scattered views of Parker

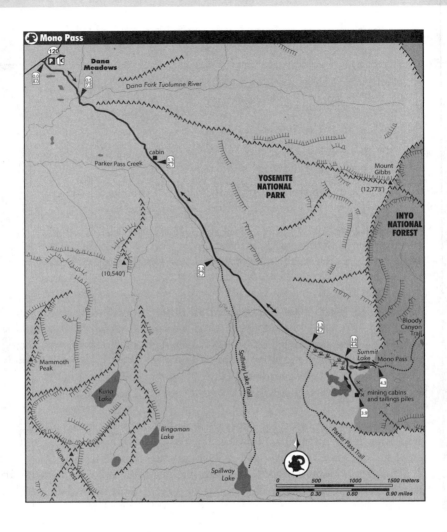

Pass Creek as you climb gently upward. Shortly you reach a junction where you will head left to Mono Pass, while the right-hand fork follows Parker Pass Creek to Spillway Lake **(2.3 miles)**. Note that the distance you have traveled is less than that indicated on most available trail maps.

Climbing more steeply now, your route diverges from Parker Pass Creek as it continues to skirt around the base of Mount Gibbs. The lodgepole pine forest is occasionally broken, yielding views to the Kuna Crest and passing one prominent rock pile. You begin to emerge from forest cover at the next trail junction **(3.3 miles)**; here you continue straight ahead to Mono Pass, while turning right takes you to Parker Pass. You are now above continuous forest cover. The slopes adjacent to the marshy stream corridor are sparsely dotted with whitebark pines, and beyond are talus mountain slopes, Mount Gibbs to the left (north) and Mount Lewis to the right (south). Continuing along the slope left (north) of the creek, you will likely see a trail crossing to the south. It leads to a collection of old mining cabins and piles of mine tailings, the piles of junk rock extracted from the mine and discarded. These are a required detour. The junction is unmarked but obvious **(3.6 miles)**.

Crossing a boggy meadow and climbing briefly through scattered whitebark pines, you pass small tailings piles and then reach five cabins **(3.9 miles)**. The cabins were built in 1879 and used for 10 years until the site was abandoned, and as with the nearby mines at Bennettville (Hike 42), little ore was ever extracted.

After returning from this side trip **(4.2 miles)**, continue toward Mono Pass and Summit Lake **(4.3 miles)**. Peering down very rugged Bloody Canyon, it is difficult to imagine that this old Native American trail was *the* route from Yosemite to the eastern Sierra until the 1880s. Today it is a little-used, very steep, and incredibly beautiful trail. Any of the lovely red rock outcrops on the slopes above the lake or the lakeshore itself make a splendid lunch location. The reddish rocks rising above Bloody Canyon, to the east, are striking. After absorbing the landscape, return to the trailhead the way you came **(8.0 miles)**.

TO THE TRAILHEAD
GPS Coordinates: N37° 53.455′ W119° 15.763′

From the Tuolumne Meadows Store, drive 5.8 miles east (toward Tioga Pass). Turn right into a small parking area. Alternatively, drive 12 miles west from the junction of US 395 and CA 120 (just south of Lee Vining by the Mobil gas station) to the Yosemite National Park boundary at the Tioga Pass entrance. Continue west an additional 1.4 miles, turning into a small parking area on the left.

39 Gaylor Lakes and Great Sierra Mine

Trailhead Location: Tioga Road at Yosemite entrance

Trail Use: Hiking

Distance & Configuration: 1.8- to 4.0-mile out-and-back

Elevation Range: 9,940 feet at the start, with a cumulative elevation change of up to ±1,250 feet

Facilities: A toilet is located at the parking lot, but the closest water is at Saddlebag Lake, in Lee Vining, or at the Tuolumne Meadows Store.

Highlights: Grassy lakeshores, views to Cathedral Range, and historic mining cabins

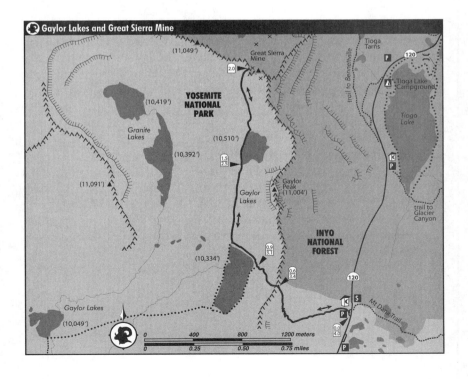

DESCRIPTION

This is a walk that has it all—as long as you are willing to ascend the steep 600 feet to the initial pass. The view across the middle Gaylor Lake to the Cathedral Range is striking: an expanse of dark-blue water with the craggy peaks as a backdrop. The meadows surrounding Gaylor Lakes are unusual for the Sierra—lush, moist grass as well as drier spots that are perfect for a picnic. If you wish to continue to the Great Sierra Mine on Tioga Hill, you can see a piece of Tioga history, including the slowly collapsing Great Sierra Cabin.

THE ROUTE

Departing from the parking area, you find the trailhead just to the southwest of the large stone toilets. The first 200 feet of climbing are moderate, taking you west through lodgepole pine forest. Wildflowers are abundant on the floor of this lush forest, especially in little grassy glades. Arriving at a steeper stretch of hillside, the trail bends to the northwest and begins climbing steeply. There are some short switchbacks, but the track is steep enough to feel as though you are heading directly upslope. Surmounting steps, roots, and simply steep inclines, take as many breathers as you need, for you are at high elevation. Enjoy the views south across an avalanche-cleared slope to Dana Meadows and Mono Pass before the trail takes you back into the forest. Take comfort in knowing that the slope will flatten in a few more switchbacks.

Leaving forest cover behind, you emerge on a dry, open saddle. The rock is a reddish color and—given that it is a dry slope—the ground is quite densely covered with small tufts of sedges (which look like short grass) and many cushion plants, low-growing alpine species that can be completely

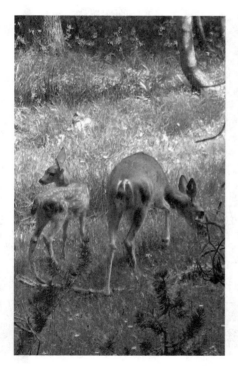
Mule deer with fawn

enveloped in colorful flowers in late June and July. A few more steps take you to the pass and a necessary vista stop **(0.6 mile from start)**. Ahead of you is the middle of the three Gaylor Lakes and behind is the large red mass of Mount Dana.

Descending nearly as steeply as you climbed, you arrive at the shores of the lake **(0.9 mile)**. Just before the lakeshore, bear right where the trail forks; heading left takes you to a fisherman's trail around the lake. The peaks that ring Tuolumne Meadows are visible in the distance. The metamorphic rocks here create a soil that can hold much more water than granitic ones do, allowing the lush flower-filled meadows (and potentially swarms of mosquitoes) to form. I am a big fan of locations where the grass extends right to the lakeshore, and much of middle Gaylor Lake is ringed by meadow. The inlet creek is likewise lush and grassy, with banks that partially curl over the stream; take care not to damage them.

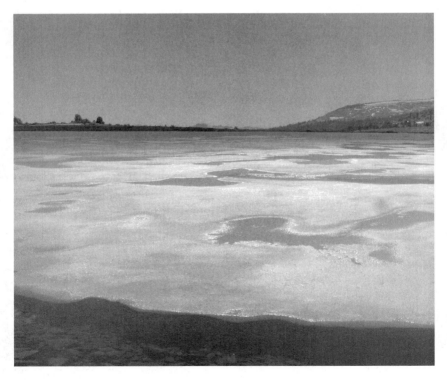

Middle Gaylor Lake still snow covered in late July

Many stop at middle Gaylor Lake, but if time and energy permit, turn right and continue to the upper Gaylor Lake and the old buildings and shafts of the Great Sierra Mine. A collection of several narrow tracks climbs through meadows beside the creek; stay in the more distinct track, even if it is a little muddy, to avoid damaging the meadow. You pass the western side of Gaylor Peak and shortly reach the upper lake, this one ringed by both meadow and scattered boulders **(1.5 miles)**. The trail continues around the left (west) side of the lake, crossing the inlet stream and then climbing upward.

Beyond, the ground becomes bare and rocky, and you climb between scattered whitebark pines. The trail leads first to an old rock cabin, the Great Sierra Cabin, missing a roof and the chimney increasingly listing. Continuing across the nearly flat landscape of rock outcrops and alpine flowers, you pass other remnants of structures, mine shafts, and tailings (junk rock) piles created during the brief, and unsuccessful, silver mining boom, 1878–1884. Exercise caution and don't explore the mine shafts. The trail ends when you reach the ridge **(2.0 miles)**. After enjoying the view, return the way you came **(4.0 miles)**.

TO THE TRAILHEAD
GPS Coordinates: N37° 54.615' W119° 15.498'
From the Tuolumne Meadows Store, drive 7.2 miles east (toward Tioga Pass), turning into a parking area left (west) of the road just before exiting the park. Alternatively, drive 12 miles west from the junction of US 395 and CA 120 (just south of Lee Vining, by the Mobil gas station), turning into a parking lot on the right (west) side of the road just after you enter Yosemite.

40 Mount Dana

Trailhead Location: Tioga Road at Yosemite entrance

Trail Use: Hiking

Distance & Configuration: 5.4-mile out-and-back

Elevation Range: 9,943 feet at the start to 13,057 feet at the summit, with 3,120 feet of ascent/descent

Facilities: A toilet is located across the street from the trailhead, but the closest water is at Saddlebag Lake, in Lee Vining, or at the Tuolumne Meadows Store.

Highlights: Rewarding views in all directions, tall rocky summit, and colorful talus

DESCRIPTION

The walk up Mount Dana, Yosemite's second-tallest peak, is a simultaneously rewarding and exhausting adventure. As you follow the use trail upward, the view becomes ever more expansive, providing good excuses to stop and catch your breath as you climb. But the view from the summit tops them all, as you stare down the vertical eastern escarpment to Mono Lake and north and south along the Sierra Crest. Do not take this walk if thunderstorms are forecast.

THE ROUTE

The unmarked trailhead lies just outside the Yosemite entrance station; follow the obvious trail straight across the tarn-dotted landscape, heading approximately east-southeast. You are following the very gentle saddle that is Tioga Pass, with the lakes to your left (north) draining to the east and those to your right (south) draining to the west. Shortly after passing two largish tarns on your left, the open meadows transition to a lodgepole pine forest. The trail bends slightly left, now trending due east as the slope increases **(0.4 mile from start)**. After a short distance the trail turns 90 degrees to the right and sidles south across the base of Mount Dana. You are now on an open slope densely covered with tall wildflowers and nicknamed Dana Gardens. Seeps and small springs allow this slope to remain moist and lush throughout the summer. The tall stalks of purple larkspurs

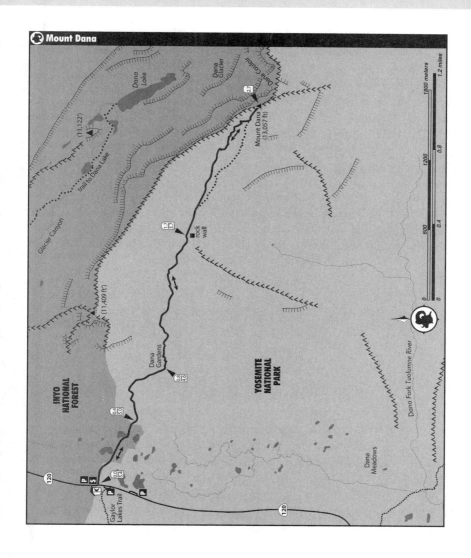

and wild onions are particularly striking. Soon the trail turns left and begins a steep climb up Mount Dana **(0.8 mile)**.

Like most unconstructed trails, this one goes nearly straight up, with only the most rudimentary switchbacks. After a 400-foot climb the continuous greenery transitions to patches of plant cover interspersed with large talus blocks, for you are now in the alpine zone where the trees are absent and the vegetation shorter. The cold winter temperatures, strong winds, and short growing season limit which species can survive.

Continuing upward at a slightly more northerly slant, the trail bends sharply right and crosses a talus tongue. The trail disappears across these rocks, but the beginning and end of this stretch are well marked by rock cairns. Marmots tend to be everywhere, sunning themselves atop large boulders. Ahead the trail angles up and across a bare slope of one of the types of red metamorphic rock that comprise Mount Dana. The rock here decomposes to small pieces, allowing a good trail to be worn by many pairs of hiking boots.

At the top of this slope you reach a broad plateau 1,700 feet above Tioga Pass **(1.7 miles)** and now have expansive views to the west, taking in Tuolumne Meadows and its surrounding peaks as well as the summits ringing Saddlebag Lake to the north. Take a well-earned rest, and then continue up across the plateau. The summit is another 1,400 feet above

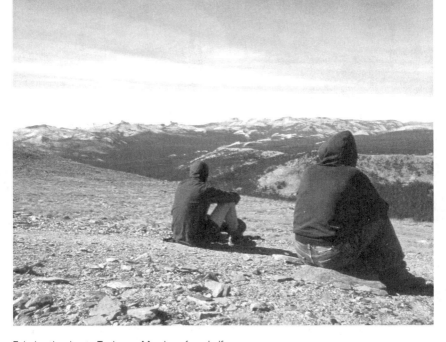

Enjoying the view to Tuolumne Meadows from halfway up

you. At least one spur trail branches to the right, but keep going in a nearly straight line, for this is the trail that remains most distinct when you enter the boulder field above.

Indeed, as you continue, the small-size substrate that was such easy walking disappears, replaced by large blocks, many with a beautiful red-purplish or greenish hue. These rocks make for more awkward strides but are beautiful to stare at. In early summer the spherical purple heads of sky pilots also entice you onward. As you climb upward, your goal is to follow the most worn path—keep your eyes focused on stripes of sand worn by earlier walkers—and accept that you will increasingly clamber over boulders when the sandy patches disappear. When in doubt, traverse a little to your right (south) or continue straight ahead. Stop often to catch your breath, drink water, and enjoy the vista.

You know you are approaching the summit when the ridges to your left and right start to converge. The trail now traverses a short distance to the right (south) before climbing the final 200 feet to the summit. The summit is broad with ample space for a long lunch (**2.7 miles**). To the northeast the face of Mount Dana drops steeply away. Beyond is Mono Lake. Other prominent summits include Mount Ritter, Mount Lyell, Cathedral Peak, and Mount Conness, but summits 60 miles to the south are visible on a clear day. If thunderclouds are building, I suggest a quick summit break and longer rest when you are below the plateau; lightning is a danger and these rocks are quite slippery when wet.

As you retrace your steps to the car (**5.4 miles**), you will no doubt question the exact path you took up the final 1,000 feet to the summit and may well select a slightly different descent—I often do—but be sure to keep the broad plateau with the windbreak wall in view to ensure that you descend the correct aspect of the mountain.

TO THE TRAILHEAD
GPS Coordinates: N37° 54.655' W119° 15.464'
From the Tuolumne Meadows Store, drive 7.2 miles east (toward Tioga Pass), parking to the right of the road just after exiting the park. Alternatively, drive 12 miles west from the junction of US 395 and CA 120 (just south of Lee Vining, by the Mobil gas station), parking on the left (east) side of the road just before you enter Yosemite. (Two parking areas are also just inside Yosemite, but the walk begins at the national park entrance.)

41 Dana Plateau

Trailhead Location: Tioga Road

Trail Use: Hiking

Distance & Configuration: 4.4- to 5.8-mile out-and-back

Elevation Range: 9,770 feet at the start to 11,680 feet at the turn-around point, with a cumulative elevation change of ±2,140 feet

Facilities: Toilets are located here, but the closest water is available at the Tuolumne Meadows Store, at Saddlebag Lake, or in Lee Vining.

Highlights: Mono Lake views, intriguing alpine tundra, and an on-top-of-the-world feel

DESCRIPTION

The enormous diversity of flowers has long made the unglaciated Dana Plateau a favorite location for Yosemite's natural history buffs, but its charm is more wide-ranging. A spring-fed trickle flows through the lower end of the slanting plateau, while its northern and eastern escarpments offer striking views of Mono Lake and Tioga Road. Giant granitic boulders dot the landscape, perfect for an afternoon nap—or marmot spotting. The generally quite good use trail becomes less distinct in a few key locations, so only choose this destination if you are comfortable with your navigation skills.

THE ROUTE

A small trail descends from the south side of the parking area and skirts around the southern edge of Tioga Lake. In the early morning you will enjoy the glassy surface of the lake and possibly a beautiful reflection of the landscape to the north, including Tioga Peak. Continuing along the grassy shore, you step across several small inlet streams. At the end of the lake, at a faint Y-junction, head straight ahead on the more prominent of the two trails; the other branch continues left along Tioga Lake's shore. In a few more steps a small sign indicates that you are on the trail to Glacier Canyon **(0.3 mile from start),** and just beyond you enter a lodgepole pine forest.

The trail switchbacks up the increasingly steep slope—switchbacks they are, but at a much steeper clip than most of the built trails in the Sierra. You cross the creek on a small log and continue your upward climb. In places the

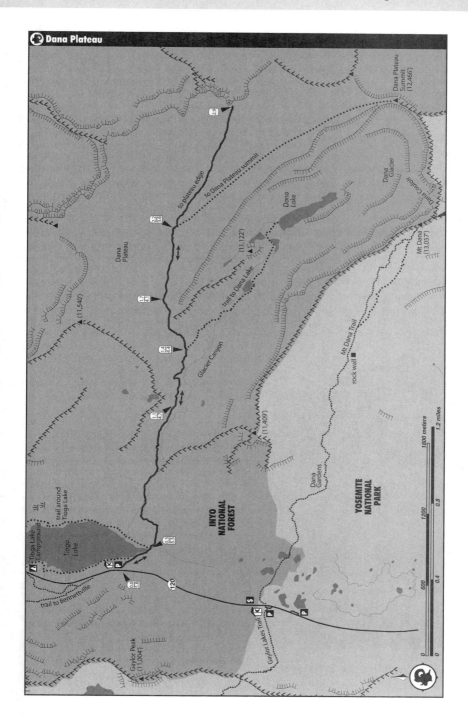

Dana Plateau

forest floor is bare and dry; elsewhere, where springs water the vegetation, you emerge from the forest cover onto lusher slopes with a colorful display of wildflowers and a touch of mud.

Just above one colorful patch the gradient eases and you reach an open bench strewn with logs from winter avalanche activity **(1.1 miles)**. After just a brief respite the trail resumes its upward trajectory, climbing up and across the slope ahead. Make sure that you are still on the north (left) side of the drainage. Where the topography next flattens, the trail bends to the left (north) and you note a marshy meadow to your right and suddenly have a wonderful view to the northwest (your left): beyond Tioga Pass lie White Mountain and Mount Conness. You now follow the trail around the western edge of the meadow, step across the small stream, and skirt to the north (left) of the marshy area. Along this section are two trails, one directly on the edge of the meadow and a second about 40 feet upslope to the north. They merge and diverge repeatedly, but both eventually climb up a short dry slope.

Now watch your step carefully as the trail seems to vanish **(1.4 miles)**. To your left, the slope turns into a broad open gully filled with small talus

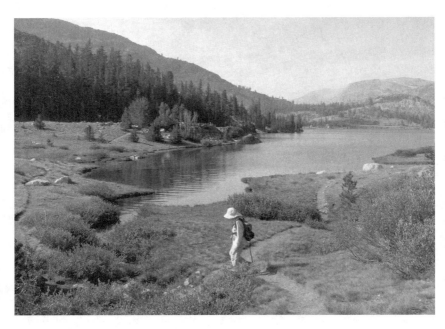

Descending to Tioga Lake at the end of the day

blocks. Straight ahead is the foot of the talus slope, followed by rolling terrain with scattered trees. Do not continue straight ahead, assuming the trail will reemerge beyond the talus. Instead, the route climbs up the left side of the talus slope. It is indistinct at the bottom, but by the time you have climbed 100 feet, the trail will reappear along the western (left) side of the slope and switchback up the slope.

At the top of the gully, the quite obvious trail bends to the right (east) and winds through a fairly flat, sandy slope covered with stunted whitebark pines **(1.7 miles)**. Beyond there are no trees, just lovely grassy meadows and a small creek. It is unusual to have a creek so high on a slope, but the gently U-shaped form of the Dana Plateau funnels moisture; on the plateau itself this results in a wonderful diversity of alpine tundra plants and denser-than-usual vegetation. The plateau was never glaciated, providing a refuge for plant species when a thick layer of ice covered all the surrounding lowlands. The trail follows the banks of the creek until quite suddenly it disappears. I consider this point the start of the Dana Plateau, for the gently sloping land that comprises the plateau suddenly expands in all directions and a trail is no longer required **(2.2 miles)**.

Once you are on the Dana Plateau you have many options for exploring. The walking is easy and fast, for the ground cover is mostly sand, grass, or small alpine herbs. Heading to the northern escarpments provides aerial views of Tioga Road and Mono Lake **(2.9 miles)**. Heading to the southern escarpment allows you to look down onto the brilliant blue waters of Dana Lake. If you have plenty of time and energy, continue straight ahead, climbing up the shallow peak at the eastern head of the plateau, for it provides views in every direction. The map indicates the route to the summit, but that distance is not included in this hike description.

Retrace your steps on the return **(5.8 miles)**. The trickiest section here is finding the top of the broad talus gully. Remember that it is beyond (west of) and to the left (south) of the slope of short scrubby whitebark pines.

TO THE TRAILHEAD

GPS Coordinates: N37° 55.258′ W119° 15.273′
From the Tuolumne Meadows Store, drive 7.2 miles east to the Yosemite boundary at Tioga Pass. Continue an additional 0.7 mile, turning into an open parking area (and vista location) to the right (east) of the road. Alternatively, drive 11.3 miles west from the junction of US 395 and CA 120 (just south of Lee Vining, by the Mobil gas station), turning left (east) into the parking area toward the southern end of and above Tioga Lake. The trail begins at the southern end of the parking area, beyond the toilets.

42 Bennettville

Trailhead Location: Tioga Road, 0.7 mile east of Yosemite National Park entrance station

Trail Use: Hiking

Distance & Configuration: 2.7-mile point to point, 4.2-mile loop, or 3.7-mile out-and-back

Elevation Range: 9,770 feet at the start to 9,520 feet at the end, with a cumulative elevation change of +170, -390

Facilities: Toilets are located here, but the closest water is available at the Tuolumne Meadows Store, Saddlebag Lake, or the Tioga Gas Mart in Lee Vining.

Highlights: Restored 1880s cabins, mining tunnel, Tioga Tarns, and flowers

DESCRIPTION

The walk past the Great Sierra Tunnel and onto Bennettville takes you back to the 1880s and Tioga Pass's brief mining boom. The subalpine setting is spectacular, with wonderful views of Mount Dana, the picturesque Tioga Tarns, and endless summer wildflowers. With such varied treats along the way and not much elevation gain, this is a perfect walk with kids.

THE ROUTE

From the trailhead, descend CA 120 a short distance to an old road on the left (east) side of the road. Continue along this road, the old Great Sierra Wagon Road, shortly reaching a junction **(0.3 mile from start)**. Bear left, first entering a small stand of trees and then emerging onto an open slope. A small creek is easily stepped across as you climb gently. The views are magnificent—Mount Dana and its sub-peak to the southeast and Tioga Peak to the northeast, all peaks of red-colored metamorphic rock. Indeed the rock underfoot is a similar color, but just a short distance west is granite, indicating that you are standing in the vicinity of a geological contact zone. Contact zones are where much mining activity occurs, for this is where metals are most likely to be concentrated.

The path takes you to the first of the Tioga Tarns, a beautiful shallow lake surrounded by verdant grass and wildflowers. Just beyond are

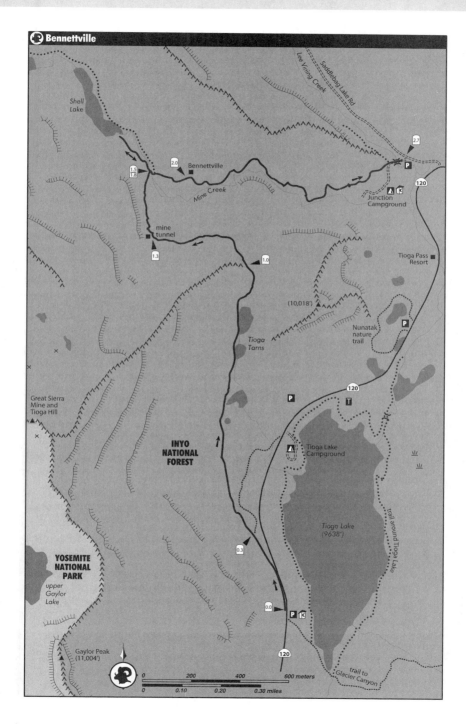

Bennettville

Shell Lake

Lee Vining Creek

Sandlebag Lake Rd

2.7

1.5
1.8

2.0 Bennettville

P

Mine Creek

120

Junction Campground

mine tunnel

1.3

1.0

Tioga Pass Resort

(10,018')

Nunatak nature trail

P

Tioga Tarns

Great Sierra Mine and Tioga Hill

120

P

T

INYO NATIONAL FOREST

Tioga Lake Campground

Tioga Lake (9638')

trail around Tioga Lake

0.3

YOSEMITE NATIONAL PARK

upper Gaylor Lake

0.0

P

Gaylor Peak (11,004')

120

trail to Glacier Canyon

0   200   400   600 meters

0   0.10   0.20   0.30 miles

two more tarns, each a bit deeper and more enclosed than the last but all picturesque and enticing should you desire a break. Climbing above the final tarn, you approach a shallow, forested saddle **(1.0 mile)** and descend into the Mine Creek drainage. Descending a dry slope, you pass a beautiful willow-lined glade densely planted with tall flowers and then see a waterfall ahead. Beyond your eyes are drawn to a large orange rock pile of mine tailings to the right and two large cabins farther to the right, the Bennettville cabins to which you are headed.

Approaching the tailings pile **(1.3 miles)**, you now see its source, a fenced-off tunnel that disappears into the mountain. This is the start of the 1,700-foot-long Great Sierra Tunnel, constructed 1882–1884 to intersect a mineral vein predicted to lie beneath Tioga Hill to your southwest. In the early spring of 1882, the impressive machinery lying around you was hauled from Lundy Canyon to the northeast, up over a very rugged ridge and to this location—it was deemed easier on snow than in summer. The following year the precursor to Tioga Road, the Great Sierra Wagon Road, was built from the west to facilitate transport to this mine. However, the mine went bankrupt before hitting any profitable veins, and like so many other mining towns, Bennettville—still a short walk ahead—went from boom to bust.

Continuing along, you traverse a dry, wildflower-covered hillside and then reach the banks of Mine Creek **(1.5 miles)**. A faint use trail departs upslope along the creek's southern bank; follow this to the outlet of Shell Lake, one of those must-see locations. Sitting on the lake's grassy shores, or on a rocky knoll just above, you can absorb views back to Mount Dana and across the lake to Mount Conness, another of Tuolumne's iconic peaks. After the requisite break, retrace your steps to the main trail **(1.8 miles)** and walk across Mine Creek on a collapsing log bridge (or unfortunately at times a wade when the log disappears).

Paralleling the creek downstream, you reach the remains of Bennettville, two large cabins that were restored in 1993 **(2.0 miles)**. During the mining boom, Bennettville was a community of many cabins, including a post office, but the others have not survived a century of winter blizzards.

From Bennettville you can return the way you came, for a total distance of 3.7 miles, or you can continue downstream, emerging at the entrance to the Junction Campground, right at the start of Saddlebag Lake Road. If you can persuade one member of your party to return for the car, a 1.5-mile walk up Tioga Road, while you eat pie at the Tioga Pass Resort, I recommend continuing down. Otherwise retrace your steps to the car. (The description continues down.)

Assuming you continue, take the time to enjoy the surrounding rocks and the narrow gorge through which Mine Creek now spills. You may have noted that creeks carved in granite are never steep-walled incised channels, but here you are still in the red metamorphic rocks. As you descend, you walk across red slabs and pass a few large granite boulders, deposited here by long-gone glaciers. After a brief climb, you see the first tents and, descending again, reach the campground **(2.7 miles)**. Cross the bridge, turn right onto Saddlebag Lake Road, cross a second bridge, and you are at CA 120. Walk uphill to your car **(4.2 miles)**.

TO THE TRAILHEAD
GPS Coordinates:
Bennettville Trailhead: N37° 55.258' W119° 15.273'
Junction Campground: N37° 56.315' W119° 15.013'
From the Tuolumne Meadows Store, drive 7.2 miles east to the Yosemite boundary at Tioga Pass. Continue an additional 0.7 mile, parking along the right side of the road at the pullout/parking lot with a vista over Tioga Lake. Alternatively, drive 11.3 miles west from the junction of US 395 and CA 120 (just south of Lee Vining, by the Mobil gas station), parking along the left-hand (east) side of the highway. To reach the ending point for this walk, continue an additional 1.5 miles down CA 120 to Saddlebag Lake Road. Turn left (north) onto Saddlebag Lake Road and turn almost immediately left into the Junction Campground. A few parking spots are at the campground entrance.

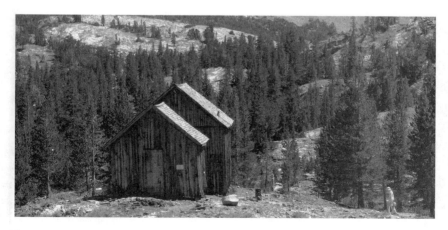

The restored Bennettville cabins

43 Gardisky Lake

Trailhead Location: Saddlebag Lake Road

Trail Use: Hiking

Distance & Configuration: 1.8-mile out-and-back

Elevation Range: 9,745 feet at the start, with 740 feet of ascent/ descent

Facilities: No amenities are located at the trailhead. The closest toilets and water are an additional 1.1 miles up Saddlebag Lake Road at the large parking area near the boat wharf.

Highlights: Bright bursts of flowers, alpine lake on a ridge, and a relaxing picnic spot

DESCRIPTION

On my many trips to Gardisky Lake, it is immediately clear that this is a hike Tuolumne area lovers return to again and again—a woman recently commented to me that she always comes here to see the wild onions blooming. Indeed, who wouldn't want to do a short hike that leads to some unbelievably dense stands of meadow wildflowers and then leads to an alpine lake that seems to be sitting on a ridge and is flanked by two easily ascended peaks?

THE ROUTE

Cross the road and begin climbing steeply through lodgepole pine forest. This trail is original in that it is a narrow path built at a high grade. It requires a bit of extra leg muscle but is very efficient and a surprisingly good walk with 5- to 10-year-old children—many kids of this age are quickly bored of walking but are quite capable of climbing up a hill. They'd much rather climb up tall steps and maneuver around tree roots than switchback for twice the distance.

You quickly reach a small creek, easily stepped across even when the water is high. Continuing up you enjoy a continuous collection of wildflowers on the dry slopes underfoot, while the willow-choked creek gurgles to the right. Eventually a sharp left-trending switchback takes you away from the creek and onto a dry slope just choked with color—red thistles, purple pennyroyals, white mariposa lilies, orange paintbrushes, and much more. You surmount the lip of the slope and the landscape flattens **(0.5 mile from start)**, revealing an expansive, slightly sloping meadow.

The creek you have been following flows down the middle, creating a wide band of wet grass and dense stands of flowers that don't mind wet feet, especially elephant's-heads and swamp onions. The grassy slopes that rise above it are drier but still colorful well into summer. Turning around yields views to White Mountain and Mount Conness. Continuing on, the topography flattens and the trail then dissipates. Bend a little to the left to reach the larger and deeper Gardisky Lake, while two shallow tarns sit to the right, lovely and warm (or already dry) in late summer. The shores of Gardisky Lake are dotted with stunted whitebark pines. In this open setting, where bitter winds whip across this slope all winter, the trees are mostly low-growing, stunted, and form beautiful shapes; they are termed krummholz, or "crooked wood."

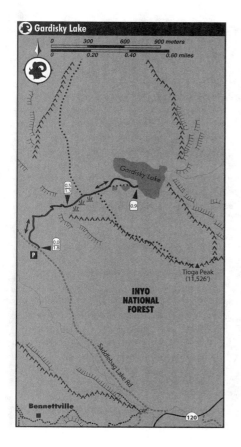

As you reach the shores of Gardisky Lake, ponder that you have just crossed a pass, for Gardisky Lake drains to the east; the creek you were following is not its outlet. This is actually a lake perched on a ridge, with views to match **(0.9 mile)**. After a quiet lunch sitting on the shores of the lake, a tarn, or the middle of a meadow, retrace your steps to the car **(1.8 miles)**.

Although the trail ends at Gardisky Lake, there are many options for continued exploration. The slope to the north is straightforward walking, providing a beautiful view of the Tioga Pass and Saddlebag Lake regions if you climb an additional 800 feet. A use trail created by hikers more or less follows the left (west) side of this slope upward. To the south lies Tioga Peak, with outstanding views to Mount Dana and into southern

Yosemite. Once above the last trees, a use trail emerges that follows the right (west) side of the face in front of you.

TO THE TRAILHEAD

GPS Coordinates: N37° 57.034' W119° 15.669'

From the Tuolumne Meadows Store, drive 9.4 miles east to the Saddle-bag Lake Road junction, en route passing the Yosemite boundary at Tioga Pass. Turn left onto Saddlebag Lake Road and continue 1.4 miles to a small parking area on the left (west) side of the road. The trailhead is directly across the road. Alternatively, drive 9.9 miles west from the junction of US 395 and CA 120 (just south of Lee Vining, by the Mobil gas station), turning right onto Saddlebag Lake Road.

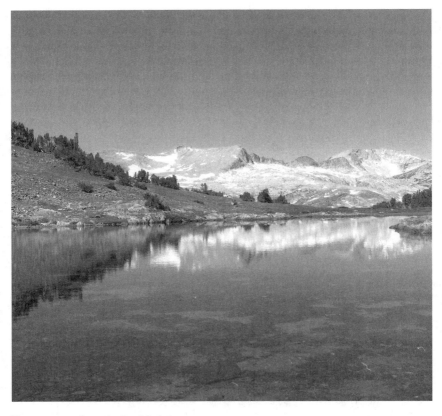

The scene west from the Gardisky Lake tarns

44 Slate Creek Fork of Lee Vining Creek

Trailhead Location: Saddlebag Lake Road

Trail Use: Hiking

Distance & Configuration: 4.2-mile out-and-back

Elevation Range: 9,780 feet at the start, with a cumulative elevation change of ±500 feet

Facilities: A toilet is available in the campground, 0.2 mile from the start. A water tap is available at Saddlebag Lake, 0.8 mile up Saddlebag Lake Road.

Highlights: Steep granite walls, shallow green meadows, and a delightfully alpine feel

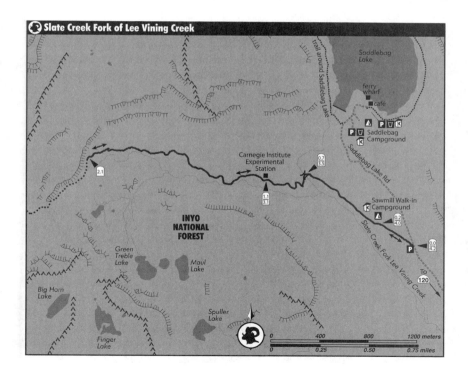

DESCRIPTION

This walk has a very different feel than most other Tioga Pass area walks, for you are not following a lake-dotted route but instead a gently sloping valley with expansive meadows interspersed with scattered groves of trees. A small creek descends the middle of the flower-filled setting. All the while you are staring at a magnificent backdrop, a semicircle of steep granite walls with year-round snowbanks. The surroundings on the entirety of this trail are so spectacular that it is satisfying to stop and sit on a beautiful rock slab anywhere beyond the Carnegie Institute cabin.

THE ROUTE

Leaving Saddlebag Lake Road, you begin by walking through the Sawmill Walk-in Campground **(0.2 mile from start)**. The track meanders past the 12 well-dispersed and picturesque campsites overlooking Lee Vining Creek and then enters a stretch of lodgepole pine forest as the trail sidles across a slope and crosses the Saddlebag Lake outlet stream on a log bridge **(0.7 mile)**.

Beyond the crossing, the trail continues beneath tree cover and shortly begins to gain elevation as it switchbacks up to a clearing, the location of the Carnegie Institute Experimental Station **(1.1 miles)**. In the 1920s this

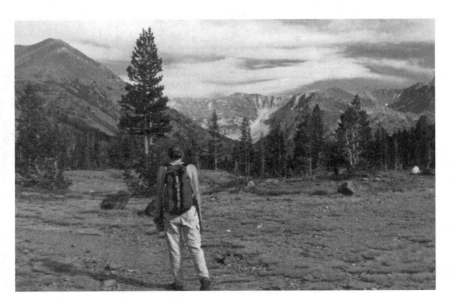

Enjoying the open vistas and flowers along the walk

station was the location of some of the first alpine plant ecology research in North America, including a famous study showing that, not surprisingly, local seeds of a species performed better than seeds of the same species from lower elevation sites. Today a few fenced areas and a cabin are indications of the location's history, but it has been little used for many decades.

It remains a wonderfully picturesque location. The steep sides of White Mountain and Mount Conness rise at the western head of the valley, while subsidiary peaks and ridges ring the basin. The headwaters of Lee Vining Creek flow through flower-filled meadows. Polished slabs stick out of these meadows, providing appealing seats. You could stop here or continue up on a well-established use trail—easy to follow because it is the route used by people climbing popular Mount Conness.

From the Carnegie Institute cabin, continue upstream, passing first through a quite marshy and flower-choked meadow and then up along the edge of the expansive meadow. As you climb, turn around for a wonderful view of the upper stretches of Lee Vining Creek with triangular, red-colored Mount Dana rising in the distance. As you climb farther, you leave behind the taller lodgepole pine forests that dominated at the trailhead and enter a landscape of scattered, stunted whitebark pines, the most common subalpine tree in Yosemite. Although this walk will not take you into the treeless true alpine zone, the whitebark pines are sufficiently sparse that the landscape of meadows, flowers, and rock has a very alpine feel.

You continue to follow a westward trajectory until the trail bends left and crosses a small, often boggy meadow (2.1 miles). Upstream (to your right), the stream is split and pours over the rock as three parallel cascades. This triplet of small waterfalls is a beautiful destination, for you have now gained enough elevation to look down upon the meadows you first passed. Granite slabs are an inviting lunch location. This is the recommended turn-around point, as beyond here, the trail becomes much less distinct. Return the way you came (4.2 miles).

TO THE TRAILHEAD
GPS Coordinates: N37° 57.340' W119° 15.968'
From the Tuolumne Meadows Store, drive 9.4 miles east to the Saddlebag Lake Road junction, en route passing the Yosemite boundary at Tioga Pass. Turn left onto Saddlebag Lake Road and continue 1.7 miles to the Sawmill Walk-in Campground; park along the roadside, leaving the campground lot for campers. Alternatively, drive 9.9 miles west from the junction of US 395 and CA 120 (just south of Lee Vining, by the Mobil gas station), turning right onto Saddlebag Lake Road.

45 Twenty Lakes Basin

Trailhead Location: Saddlebag Lake Road

Trail Use: Hiking

Distance & Configuration: 4.4-mile loop

Elevation Range: 10,066 feet at the start, with a cumulative elevation change of ±750 feet

Facilities: Toilets and a water tap are available in the parking lot.

Highlights: Countless lakes, tall escarpments, and beautiful flowers in an enormous basin

DESCRIPTION

This is the ultimate location hike, for every step of the route is beautiful. You pass seven named lakes and many more unnamed tarns. The steep northern faces of Mount Conness and North Peak are visible much of the way, and flowers are abundant throughout. This makes it a good walk with young kids because you will have had a stunning walk even if you don't complete the circuit.

THE ROUTE

This hike begins by taking the Saddlebag Lake ferry to the lake's northern shore. You book your ferry ticket at the restaurant on the lake's edge. But a word of warning: The ferries fill up very quickly in the morning, so expect at least an hour's wait at the ferry dock after you purchase your ticket. As you pick a time for your return ferry, note that you should allow 5 hours for this walk, even though it is short in distance, for part of the trail is slow walking, you are at high elevation, and you of course want ample time for breaks. (You can include the walk around Saddlebag Lake in your hike, but this adds 3 miles to your day.)

From the northern ferry wharf, take the left-hand (northwesterly) fork. As you walk along the old mining road, you will quickly realize why this is a location hike: everywhere are flowers, peaks, and water in a superb subalpine setting. Continue straight ahead at an X-junction, passing around the northern tip of Greenstone Lake. A distinct left-hand bend **(0.9 mile from start)** lies just beyond an easily overlooked pass. Beyond

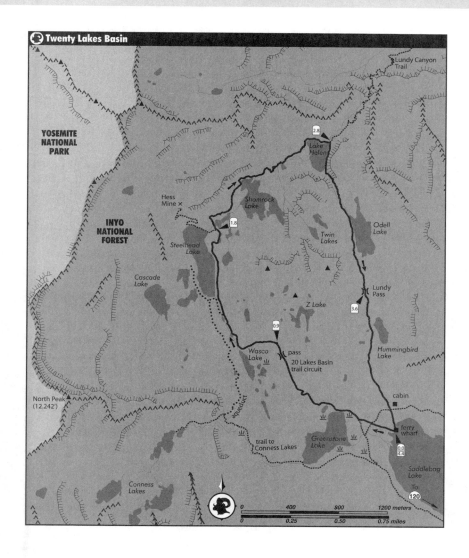

this point the water drains north and then east, flowing into Mill Creek in Lundy Canyon. The landscape is now dry with scattered whitebark pines, but flowers are abundant and varied; some species require the marshy meadows and others thrive on the dry sandy slopes. With a good plant book in hand, you will find 50 species. You next pass long, skinny Wasco Lake and then several tarns, often filled with tadpoles.

Continuing north, you reach the expansive, deep, and very intense blue waters of Steelhead Lake. A side trail branches off at its inlet, leading to lovely granite slabs above the western shores of the lake, a possible shorter destination. The trail, however, follows the eastern edge of this lake, one of the few lakeshores on this walk without good play spots, for its waters deepen rapidly at the shore. It is, however, an excellent location for fishing. Toward the end of the lake, you climb briefly between smooth outcrops and pass two inviting tarns before descending back to Steelhead Lake's outlet. The trail steps across the creek **(1.8 miles)**, and you leave the good trail and instead follow a less-engineered route northeast. (Indeed, the road now zigzags up to Hess Mine, one of the many old mines in the region. Look at the landscape and notice that you are close to the boundary—or contact—between the older red metamorphic and younger granitic rocks, the geologic setting in which metals tend to accumulate and where mines are located.)

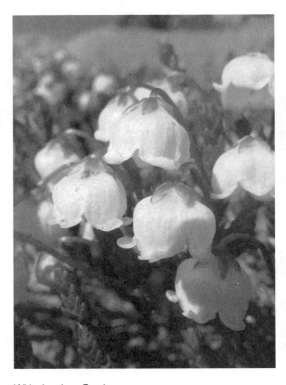

White heather, *Cassiope*

The route from this stream crossing to Lake Helen follows a well-worn use trail. It is mostly quite obvious, but in sections it disappears where steep slabs block straight-ahead progress. Cairns, rock piles placed by others, always indicate the best way ahead; if the terrain becomes steep, hunt for these markers, indicating a safe way to scramble down the slabs. It also helps to always have your eyes on the trail ahead, usually quite obvious, so you know where you should end up at the base of the slabs. The trail is the least distinct as you descend below Shamrock Lake but again emerges distinctly on a short talus slope as you approach Lake Helen.

Clamoring down to and stepping across Lake Helen's outlet, you reach a T-junction **(2.8 miles)**. Turning left takes you down to Lundy Canyon, while you will head right to complete your circuit. At this point, take the time to look west to Mount Conness and North Peak; it is a beautiful view of these peaks' steep north faces, at times reflected in Lake Helen. Now facing south, you walk up a lovely little gully, often thick with white columbines, toward Odell Lake. You climb onto a dry slope above the lake, meandering past wildflowers and occasional trees to the gentle Lundy Pass **(3.6 miles)**. Beyond the pass you descend gradually to meadows and quite shallow Hummingbird Lake. This is another location to enjoy the view of the steep Sierra Crest. And after a short stretch of forest, you reach Saddlebag Lake and can sit down and wait for the ferry back to your car **(4.4 miles)**.

TO THE TRAILHEAD

GPS Coordinates: N37° 58.839' W119° 17.053'

From the Tuolumne Meadows Store, drive 9.4 miles east to the Saddlebag Lake Road junction, en route passing the Yosemite boundary at Tioga Pass. Turn left onto Saddlebag Lake Road and continue 2.5 miles to the end of the road and park in the roadside lot that overlooks Saddlebag Lake. It is just beyond the campground entrance. To the north are the ferry wharf and restaurant where you buy your ferry ticket. Alternatively, drive 9.9 miles west from the junction of US 395 and CA 120 (just south of Lee Vining, by the Mobil gas station), turning right onto Saddlebag Lake Road.

46 Conness Lakes

Trailhead Location: Saddlebag Lake Road

Trail Use: Hiking

Distance & Configuration: 5.2-mile out-and-back

Elevation Range: 10,085 feet at the start to 10,545 feet at the turnaround point, with a cumulative elevation change of ±610 feet

Facilities: Toilets and a water tap are available in the parking lot.

Highlights: Vibrant aqua-colored glacial lakes, verdant meadows, and an aqueduct from the mining days

DESCRIPTION

This is another of the region's striking destinations. One can spend a long lunch staring at the intense glacial aqua color of Conness Lakes set against smooth granite slabs. And the walk from Saddlebag Lake is engaging—flower-filled and surrounded by the steep granite walls of Mount Conness and North Peak. An added bonus is walking beside a historic aqueduct that leads from below the Conness Lakes to Wasco Lake.

THE ROUTE

From the Saddlebag Lake parking area, cross the road, retrace your path a few feet down Saddlebag Lake Road, and descend along a closed dirt road that leads toward the base of the dam. Continuing up the other side of the gully, you will soon be on the western edge of the dam and the start of the trail that circumnavigates Saddlebag Lake **(0.2 mile from start)**. You traverse the western lakeshore on the nearly flat trail, climbing just slightly as you cross in and out of talus fans that have poured down from the slopes above. Scan the lake's deep-blue waters and the skies overhead for California gulls and perhaps even an osprey.

When the slope to your left ends, you enter a section of marshy meadows and note an unmarked trail departing to your left; this is the best route to Conness Lakes **(1.3 miles)**. If you took the ferry across the lake, from the ferry wharf, head 0.4 mile counterclockwise around Saddlebag Lake to this location. The route continues around the southern side of Greenstone Lake, through a grassy landscape scattered with boulders and striped by repeated

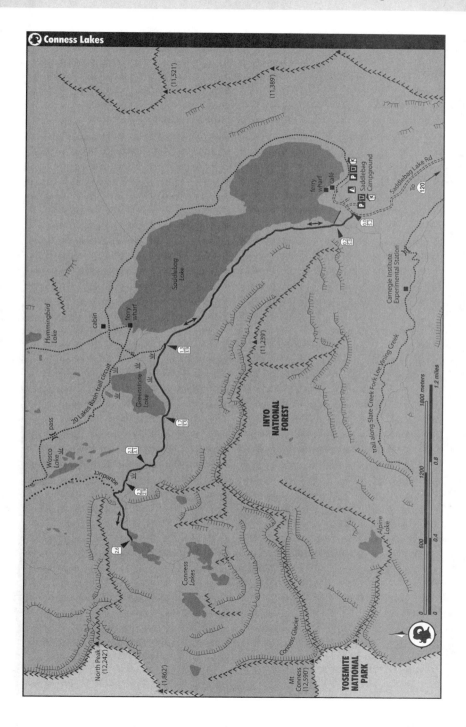

trickles of water, making this a marshy walk in early summer. Take care to stay on the trail, even when muddy, instead of eroding additional trails. Enjoy the never-ending flowers, especially the alpine asters, elephant's-heads, and red heather as you approach the Greenstone Lake inlet and a cluster of willow shrubs. Although the track appears to continue upstream, it is best to cross here on boulders just upstream of the lake inlet **(1.7 miles)**.

Now following the creek's north side, you continue through the meadows before the trail bends to the right and begins a steeper ascent. After a short, but notably steep, climb through a stand of whitebark pines, you reach another grassy bench **(2.1 miles)**. Ahead you note an abrupt increase in the slope of the terrain—there are waterfalls and no obvious route. The

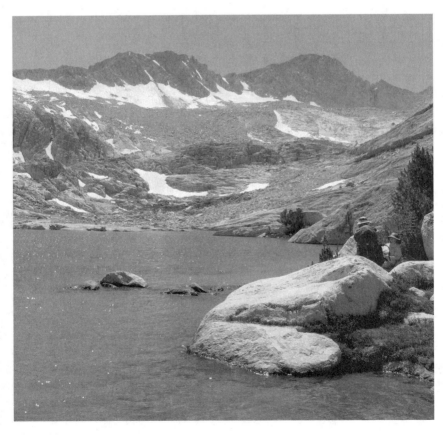

The lower Conness Lake and Mount Conness

trail indeed becomes less distinct and diverges a little from the watercourse at the end of the meadow. Looking up to the right of the falls, you will note a section of talus and then a stretch of quite bare slab. As you continue up, you'll see that the trail is easily discerned through the talus but seems to end at the slab. It sneaks nearly unnoticed to the right of the slab and later traverses above the top of the slab.

The trail climbs another 40 feet and then bends left (west), back toward the creek. You are now following a nearly flat trajectory and note the trail is again distinct **(2.3 miles)**. In fact, you are now walking beside an old aqueduct built during the mining era to carry water toward Steelhead Lake. In stretches, the rockwork is still intact. Above you will see one steeper slope—the final climb before the lakes. There are several trails—one farther left that weaves in and out of streamside vegetation and one to the right, climbing a steep dry slope next to a rock outcrop. Pick your choice, for they both lead over a lip and into the Conness Lakes basin.

Once more on the flat, you are now crossing alpine meadow and smooth granite slabs. Within minutes you come upon the first large lake (10,543 feet) and will plop yourself down to sun on beautiful granite rock, much like a marmot **(2.6 miles)**. Return the way you came **(5.2 miles)**. Or if you wish to further explore the basin, cross the outlet of this lake, and continue around its southern shore before following the inlet stream up (and south) to a lake at 10,664 feet. Each of the lakes has a subtly different color, for more glacial flour is present in the higher lakes.

TO THE TRAILHEAD

GPS Coordinates: N37° 57.953' W119° 16.305'

From the Tuolumne Meadows Store, drive 9.4 miles east to the Saddlebag Lake Road junction, en route passing the Yosemite boundary at Tioga Pass. Turn left onto Saddlebag Lake Road and continue 2.4 miles to nearly the road's end. Park in the hiker parking area—the first parking lot you encounter and before the campground entrance. Alternatively, drive 9.9 miles west from the junction of US 395 and CA 120 (just south of Lee Vining, by the Mobil gas station), turning right onto Saddlebag Lake Road. If you plan to take the ferry across (making the round-trip walk 1.8 miles shorter), continue past the campground entrance to a large parking area and purchase your ticket from the restaurant above the ferry wharf.

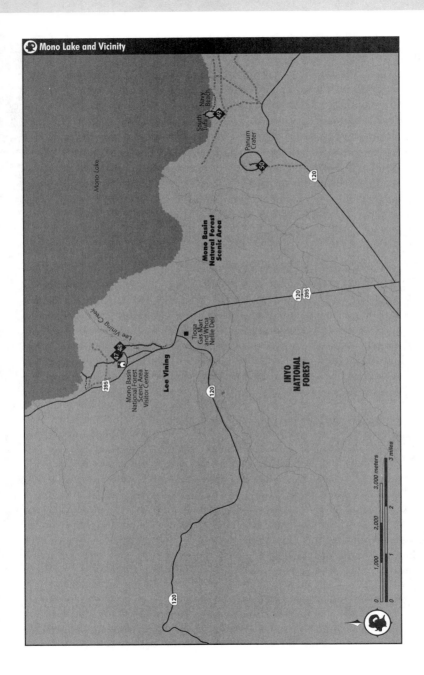

Mono Lake and Vicinity

MONO LAKE AND VICINITY

Regional Overview

The Mono Basin lies 12 road miles east of and 3,000 feet in elevation below Tioga Pass, the eastern entrance to Yosemite National Park. Mono Lake, most visitors' focus, is a large salt lake at its center. The lake has been made famous both by its fantastic tufa towers, tall calcium carbonate statues decorating stretches of lakeshore and shallow waters, and the fact that its source streams have been diverted by Los Angeles since 1941. This diversion lowered the lake level and led to a well-known legal battle that fortunately led to a decrease in water diversions and partial refilling of the lake.

Consider a visit to Mono Lake and the adjacent town of Lee Vining if you are accessing Yosemite from the east or if you have an extended time in Tuolumne Meadows and wish to venture farther afield for a day. The lake is especially stunning in early morning and evening light, most notably during or after a thunderstorm.

Many excellent walks are also located in the nearby canyons, but here I include only a selection of four short walks on or near the shores of Mono Lake. Young children can easily complete three of the walks, while the fourth, Panum Crater (Hike 50), involves more elevation gain and an arduous, but very worthwhile, slog up volcanic cinder. South Tufa (Hike 49) is the first destination a newcomer to Mono Lake should visit. The tufa towers against a backdrop of blue lake and sky are exquisite. The walk from the visitor center to the lake's shore (Hike 47) provides more solitude and stunning lake views but only small tufa towers. Lee Vining Creek (Hike 48) is a chance to see the often-overlooked freshwater face of the Mono Basin and is beautiful in October when the tree leaves are yellow.

In summer the Mono Basin is hot and dry, so wear sun hats, apply sunscreen, and carry water for even the shortest excursions. I often feel more worn out after a touristy exploration of the tufa towers than following a much longer hike around Tuolumne Meadows because I have forgotten to properly outfit myself.

No visit to Mono Lake is complete without a quick stop at the Mono Basin National Forest Scenic Area Visitor Center at the northern end of Lee Vining, with excellent displays on the lake's unique ecosystem. The Mono Lake Committee Bookstore in the middle of Lee Vining is also exceptional.

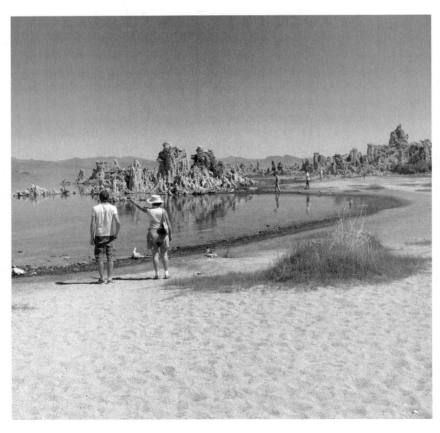

The shoreline at South Tufa (see page 215)

47 Lee Vining Visitor Center to Mono Lake

Trailhead Location: Mono Basin National Forest Scenic Area Visitor Center

Trail Use: Hiking, accessible to all-terrain strollers

Distance & Configuration: 2.8-mile out-and-back

Elevation Range: 6,705 feet at the start, with 320 feet of descent/ascent

Facilities: Toilets and water are available at the visitor center.

Highlights: Mono Lake views, boardwalk, and tufa towers

DESCRIPTION

This easy walk boasts beautiful views of Mono Lake, a cold tufa cave you can enter, and a boardwalk leading through wetlands to the shores of Mono Lake. Placards provide background information of the region's vegetation and human history. This walk is accessible year-round, excluding particularly snowy winter periods.

THE ROUTE

This recently constructed trail departs from the northwest side of the Mono Basin National Forest Scenic Area Visitor Center, also known as the Lee Vining Visitor Center, behind the big information panels in the courtyard. A few sections have been newly built, and elsewhere preexisting dirt roads are being partially revegetated to create a narrower trail, better suited for walking. Initially you are on a nature trail that leads to the back of the visitor center, but almost immediately you branch off to the left (north), descending to a beautiful bench and vista spot **(0.1 mile from start).**

The next stretch of trail is the steepest, with two short sections of stairs, but still navigable with a rugged stroller and determined parent. You are passing through a landscape of gray-green–leaved desert shrubs, which transforms into a brightly colored landscape in late spring (when the pink-colored desert peach blooms) or fall (when the yellow rabbitbrush and sagebrush bloom). On this slope the shrubs must tolerate lots of sun and little water, but conditions are even harsher on the plain below: there the soils are exceedingly salty and even fewer plants can establish.

Where the trail intersects a dirt road **(0.6 mile)**, continue straight ahead beyond a large information sign. Continuing down the slope, you reach a solo tufa tower. Take a detour inside to enjoy the cooler temperatures. Indeed, early pioneers used this location for cold storage.

The trail next intersects a boardwalk **(1.2 miles)**, built in memory of David Gaines, the founder of the Mono Lake Committee. You turn right, following the boardwalk toward Mono Lake's shore. This allows you to cross on top of a salt marsh habitat, enjoying the tall reeds with dry shoes and without impacting the vegetation.

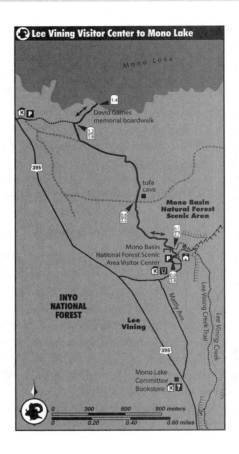

Where the boardwalk ends, you are a short distance from the lakeshore **(1.4 miles)**. Feel free to walk the last stretch to the lakeshore, feeling the rough tufa, watching masses of squirming brine shrimp, and startling the alkali flies densely lining the water's edge. Return the way you came **(2.8 miles)**. If you wish to learn more about these creatures, visit the visitor center (where you parked your car) after your walk.

You will note that on the map, the trail does not reach Mono Lake's shore, for the water level has risen since the map from which the lake's shape was adopted was published. As outlined by a landmark agreement with the Los Angeles Department of Water and Power, it will continue to rise, ensuring the lake's two islands, Negit and Paoha, remain safe bird breeding

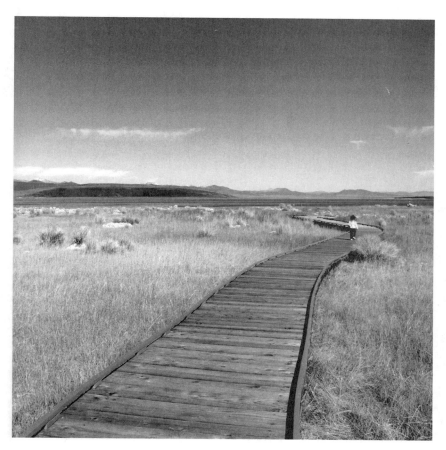

David Gaines Memorial Boardwalk

grounds, that a ring of salty dust doesn't surround the lake, and that the inlet streams boast healthy riparian habitats.

TO THE TRAILHEAD

GPS Coordinates: N37° 57.978' W119° 7.245'

From the junction of US 395 and CA 120 (just south of Lee Vining, by the Mobil gas station), drive 1.2 miles north through Lee Vining (on US 395). A large sign indicates the turnoff for the Mono Basin National Forest Scenic Area Visitor Center. Drive 0.3 mile down the unnamed spur road to a large parking area.

48 Lee Vining Creek

Trailhead Location: Mono Basin National Forest Scenic Area Visitor Center

Trail Use: Hiking

Distance & Configuration: 2.2-mile out-and-back

Elevation Range: 6,705 feet at the start, with a cumulative elevation change of ±200 feet

Facilities: Toilets and water are available at the visitor center.

Highlights: Aspen glades, banks of bubbling Lee Vining Creek, and Mono Lake views

DESCRIPTION

If you wish to see Mono Lake from a new perspective, this is a wonderful little walk, especially when the aspens are colorful or on a winter day when you wish to look down upon Mono Lake from above. This path descends through the sagebrush scrub to the banks of Lee Vining Creek and then follows the creek upstream toward the northern end of Lee Vining. This walk is accessible year-round, excluding particularly snowy winter periods.

THE ROUTE

The trailhead is located at a small opening in the rock wall along the back (east) perimeter of the visitor center. A small sign indicates the start of the trail. Turn right (south) and walk across the sagebrush, enjoying the views of Mono Lake 350 feet below you. Imagine how different the Mono Basin looked in the past: the lake was 35 feet higher before the city of Los Angeles began water diversions. More difficult to imagine, during the ice age 100,000 year ago, the lake level was 800 feet higher than today, placing your current location under hundreds of feet of water. As you begin your walk, you will notice the Lee Vining Creek course incised deeply to the southeast—a broad tree-dotted corridor lying below the dry scrubby bluffs that you are on. The well-watered stream banks are essential to the local wildlife, for the waters of Mono Lake are too salty to drink, and the animals became scarce when water diversions stopped creeks from flowing into Mono Lake. Both placards along the trail and the visitor center provide additional information on the regeneration of Lee Vining Creek and nearby waterways.

The trail follows an approximately southward trajectory as it winds down the escarpment to the riverbank. Along the final slope, the vegetation changes quite suddenly as the gray-green leaves of sagebrush, rabbitbrush, and other dry-site species give way to thickets of roses and tall trees. The roses sport dainty pink flowers in spring and have leaves that turn a rich auburn in fall. In the direction of the lake, cottonwoods dominate, while quaking aspens are common farther upstream—the latter's leaves are more richly colored in fall. Once at creek level **(0.6 mile from start)**, the trail follows the bank upstream, at times in moister riparian vegetation and elsewhere diverging back into drought-tolerant shrubs. Along this open section, there are several locations for a picnic beside the rushing creek. Up

ahead and to your right (west), you can see a row of houses and realize that you are parallel to Lee Vining.

Continuing upstream, you shortly reenter a dense aspen forest. During a few weeks in fall, the forest floor is carpeted with bright yellow leaves, and occasionally an early cold snap can even cause them to turn a vibrant orange. Enjoy this location from a well-situated bench in the middle of a stand of trees.

Just after you exit the grove of aspens, you reach a trail junction. The right-hand (west) fork is the continuation of the Lee Vining Creek Trail, while straight ahead is a less-used trail that continues along the creek **(1.1 miles)**. When you reach this junction, turn around and retrace your steps to the visitor center **(2.2 miles)**. If some members of your party wish to take a shorter walk, you are only 5 minutes from the southern end of Lee Vining. From the just-described junction, the Lee Vining Creek Trail bends right and climbs a few switchbacks to US 395. You ascend the final stretch below a large retaining wall and suddenly find yourself staring at the Lakeview Lodge.

TO THE TRAILHEAD

GPS Coordinates: N37° 58.034' W119° 7.195'

From the junction of US 395 and CA 120 (just south of Lee Vining, by the Mobil gas station), drive 1.2 miles north through Lee Vining (on US 395). Here a large sign indicates the turnoff for the Mono Basin National Forest Scenic Area Visitor Center. Drive 0.3 mile down the unnamed spur road to a large parking area.

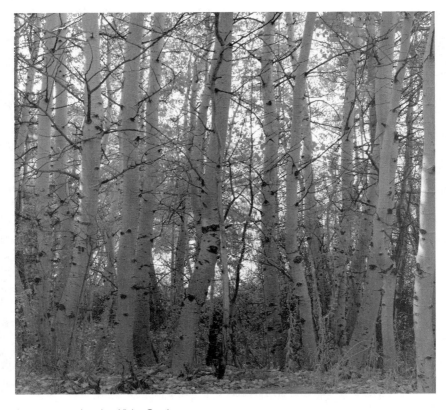

Aspen groves along Lee Vining Creek

49 South Tufa

Trailhead Location: CA 120, 5 miles east of US 395

Trail Use: Hiking

Distance & Configuration: 0.9-mile loop

Elevation Range: 6,405 feet at the start, with 20 feet of descent/ascent

Facilities: Toilets are located at the trailhead. The closest water is at the Tioga Gas Mart, the Mono Lake Committee Bookstore, and the Mono Basin National Forest Scenic Area Visitor Center.

Highlights: California gulls atop tufa towers and vibrant blues

DESCRIPTION

A visit to South Tufa is a requirement for every Yosemite-area tourist and hiker. This is certainly not a long walk, and in summer it is hot and crowded, but it is an absolutely unique location to experience. The odd-shaped tufa towers projecting skyward, the thick bands of alkali flies swarming the shores, and the expansive blue water and bright-blue skies all capture visitor's imaginations. Children are especially drawn to the birds and flies along the shore.

THE ROUTE

The loop walk departs from behind the kiosk—don't forget to pay the fees—and heads down a paved trail toward Mono Lake. You are passing through a collection of salt-tolerant vegetation, for the soils here were submerged 60 years ago and are still very salty.

Ahead you see the first tufa towers, an unnatural "natural world" attraction, for they are visible (above water) mostly due to humans diverting water from Mono Lake for Los Angeles's water supply, lowering the lake level. Tufa towers form underwater when water from calcium-rich underground springs intersects the carbonate-rich water of Mono Lake, forming calcium carbonate, or limestone. The tufa towers you are now admiring are no longer being added to, since they are no longer submerged. Signs along the trail indicate the lake's pre-diversion level and the level to which the lake has been legally mandated to refill. Shortly you reach the lakeshore **(0.3 mile from start)** and additional information signs about the lake's unusual ecosystem. From here, detour along the lakeshore, wandering up to (but not on to) the tufa towers, letting your children chase the thick stripe of alkali flies along the water's edge, admiring the brine shrimp, and taking photos of California gulls squawking from atop the towers.

When you are finished, note a sign and a trail just next to it departing to the left (east) of where you first reached the lakeshore **(0.5 mile, including detour among towers)**. Follow this trail through the scrub, passing additional information placards as you weave between tufa towers. To the east is a less-visited but often mucky stretch of shoreline. Here is a wonderful place from which to observe some of the many birds that are

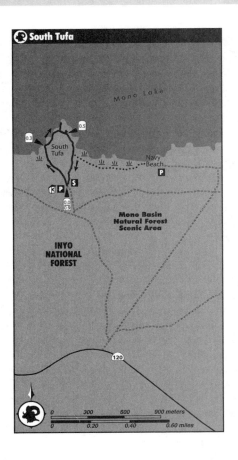

seasonal visitors to Mono Lake. The trail bends farther right, eventually heading back to the parking area **(0.9 mile)**. If you have time, a visit to the Mono Basin National Forest Scenic Area Visitor Center, northeast of Lee Vining, is recommended.

TO THE TRAILHEAD

GPS Coordinates: N37° 56.344' W119° 1.625'
From the junction of US 395 and CA 120 (just south of Lee Vining, by the Mobil gas station), drive 4.7 miles south on US 395. Now turn left (east) onto the continuation of CA 120. Drive for 4.7 miles, turning left (north) onto a road signposted for South Tufa. Bear left at a junction after 0.1 mile, continuing a total of 1 mile to a parking lot.

50 Panum Crater

Trailhead Location: CA 120, 3 miles east of US 395

Trail Use: Hiking

Distance & Configuration: 0.7-mile out-and-back or 2.1-mile loop and spur

Elevation Range: 6,830 feet at the start, with a cumulative elevation change of up to ±600 feet

Facilities: No amenities are located at the trailhead. The closest water is at the Tioga Gas Mart, the Mono Lake Committee Bookstore, and the Mono Basin National Forest Scenic Area Visitor Center. Toilets are available at the South Tufa parking area.

Highlights: Obsidian blocks, Mono Lake views, and volcanic sand

DESCRIPTION

Panum Crater is a cinder cone that rises from the expanse of sagebrush near the southwestern edge of Mono Lake. Walking around the caldera rim provides exquisite views of Mono Lake, especially in the late afternoon and evening, while the middle of the cone lets you admire jagged volcanic rock. Beware that the loop around the crater rim is a lot more difficult than it appears because you climb up long sandy slopes three times, with your shoes sinking into the soft substrate and slipping backward with each step. However, the views of Mono Lake are well worth the effort. This walk is accessible year-round, excluding particularly snowy winter periods. Also avoid it midday on hot summer days.

THE ROUTE

Departing from the parking area, you walk past an information sign and begin climbing up a broad trail of volcanic sand, slipping a little backward with each step. At a junction **(0.1 mile from start)**, the left fork takes you to the center of the cone, while straight ahead is the Rim Trail. Begin by branching to the left, traversing north across a cinder slope and then following switchbacks upward. Notice how sparse the vegetation is, for few species—even drought-tolerant desert shrubs—can survive on these coarse, exceedingly dry volcanic sands. As you ascend you will scoff at the signs reminding you to follow the established track, for walking is already such tough work that no one could want to ascend a steeper grade, but do remember to respect the landscape on your return.

The well-delineated trail ends among a jumble of tall volcanic rocks **(0.35 mile)**. Bend over to feel them, noting how smooth some surfaces are, yet how abrasive the edges are. The soles of shoes wear out quickly when traversing these rocks. From here you have a broken vista to Mono Lake and can see the Rim Trail to the east. Despite the many use trails in its direction, do not be tempted to head cross-country toward the rim, for the deep crater lies between you and this destination. Other use trails trend north along rocks; these are pleasant walking and fun to explore, but you never obtain an open view to the lake, for there are always more outcrops of volcanic rock to negotiate.

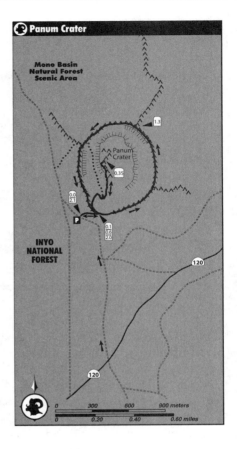

Instead, retrace your steps toward the parking area, going as far as the T-junction **(0.6 mile)**, and turn left onto the Rim Trail (right heads 0.1 mile to your car). Your route is now a nearly perfect circle, staying exactly on the crater's ridge as it undulates up (and down) to three high points. The views of Mono Lake and the Mono Basin are ever changing—broadest when you are highest but always beautiful and encompassing you as you walk. After much effort you reach the second and highest summit **(1.3 miles)**. Take a long break to enjoy your surroundings before descending steeply to a notch. So much effort to climb the slope and so easy to race down!

At the notch after the highest summit, there are several trail options. The left-most trail ascends a narrow gully, straight ahead continues along the crater's rim (and is the option described here), and heading right leads you to a dirt road west of the crater (and eventually to the parking lot). As you continue along the rim, you have an excellent view of the rocky crater center and of the broad braided flood plains to the southwest. The Rim Trail you are following eventually intersects the main trail near the previously described T-junction **(2.0 miles)**. Turn right and descend to your car **(2.1 miles)**.

TO THE TRAILHEAD
GPS Coordinates: N37° 55.538' W119° 2.925'
From the junction of US 395 and CA 120 (just south of Lee Vining, by the Mobil gas station), drive 4.7 miles south on US 395. Now turn left (east) onto the continuation of CA 120. Drive for 3.1 miles, turning left (north) onto a gravel road for the final 0.9 mile to the parking area. Do not be tempted to take unmarked dirt roads in this region.

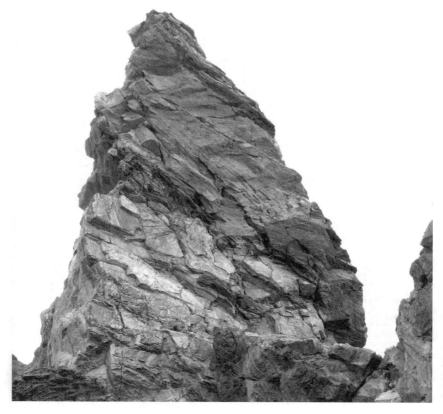

A spire of volcanic rock atop Panum Crater

HIKES AT A GLANCE

REGION / Hike # Hike name	page	hike mileage	stroller accessible	summits	<200' elevation gain	200-500' elevation gain	very short walk	swimming	use trail	winter accessible (usually)	lakes	waterfalls	vista point	sequoia groves
HETCH HETCHY RESERVOIR														
1 Lookout Point	18	2.8			X									
2 Poopenaut Valley	22	2.4						X		X				
3 Wapama Falls	25	4.8								X		X		
YOSEMITE VALLEY														
4 Base of El Capitan	34	0.8					X		X	X				
5 Bridalveil Falls	37	0.8	X		X		X			X		X		
6 Upper Yosemite Fall	40	6.4										X	X	
7 Lower Yosemite Fall	46	1.2	X		X					X		X		
8 Swinging Bridge and Superintendent's Bridge	50	2.0	X		X					X		X		
9 Mirror Lake	54	3.4			X			X		X				
10 Base of Vernal Fall	58	2.2	X							X		X		
11 Mist Trail and Clark Point	63	2.8–6.2										X	X	
GLACIER POINT ROAD AND WAWONA														
12 McGurk Meadow	71	2.0			X									
13 Taft Point	75	2.4			X								X	
14 Sentinel Dome	79	2.2		X										
15 Glacier Point	83	0.6	X		X		X					X	X	
16 Four Mile Trail	86	4.8										X	X	
17 Panorama Trail	91	8.2										X	X	
18 Lower Chilnualna Falls	96	0.7			X							X		
19 Wawona Meadow	99	3.6			X					X				
20 Mariposa Grove	102	4.9												X

HIKES AT A GLANCE

REGION Hike # Hike name		page	hike mileage	stroller accessible	summits	<200' elevation gain	200–500 elevation gain	very short walk	swimming	use trail	winter accessible (usually)	lakes	waterfalls	vista point	sequoia groves
TIOGA ROAD AND TENAYA LAKE															
21	Merced Grove	109	3.2												X
22	Crane Flat Lookout	112	0.4		X	X		X							
23	Tuolumne Grove	115	2.7	X			X								X
24	Lukens Lake (from White Wolf)	118	4.6				X					X			
25	May Lake	122	2.9				X					X		X	
26	Mount Hoffmann	125	5.8		X					X		X			
27	Olmsted Point	129	0.5		X	X		X							
28	Tenaya Lake	132	2.9			X			X			X			
TUOLUMNE MEADOWS															
29	Pothole Dome	139	1.4		X		X			X					
30	Tuolumne River	142	3.2			X			X	X					
31	Lower Cathedral Lake	145	7.4									X			
32	Cathedral Peak Shoulder	149	5.4							X				X	
33	Elizabeth Lake	153	4.2									X			
34	Soda Springs and Tuolumne Meadows	156	1.8–1.9			X									
35	Dog Lake	160	2.4–3.6						X			X			
36	Lembert Dome	163	2.4		X										
37	Lyell Canyon	166	1.6–7.6			X									

HIKES AT A GLANCE

REGION / Hike # Hike name	page	hike mileage	stroller accessible	summits	< 200' elevation gain	200–500' elevation gain	very short walk	swimming	use trail	winter accessible (usually)	lakes	waterfalls	vista point	sequoia groves
TIOGA PASS														
38 Mono Pass	173	8.0									X			
39 Gaylor Lakes and Great Sierra Mine	176	1.8–4.0									X		X	
40 Mount Dana	180	5.4		X					X					
41 Dana Plateau	184	4.4–5.8							X				X	
42 Bennettville	188	2.7–4.2				X					X		X	
43 Gardisky Lake	192	1.8									X		X	
44 Slate Creek Fork of Lee Vining Creek	195	4.2				X			X				X	
45 Twenty Lakes Basin	198	4.4									X			
46 Conness Lakes	202	5.2							X		X		X	
MONO LAKE AND VICINITY														
47 Lee Vining Visitor Center to Mono Lake	209	2.8	X			X				X	X		X	
48 Lee Vining Creek	212	2.2			X					X			X	
49 South Tufa	215	0.9	X		X					X	X	X		
50 Panum Crater	217	0.7–2.1		X						X				

INDEX

About the Author

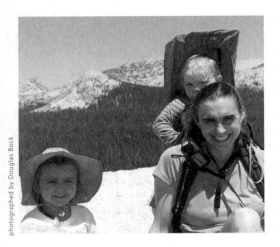

photographed by Douglas Bock

Since childhood, Elizabeth "Lizzy" Wenk has hiked and climbed in the Sierra Nevada with her family. After she started college, she found excuses to spend every summer in the Sierra, with its beguiling landscape, abundant flowers, and near-perfect weather. During those summers, she worked as a research assistant for others and completed her own Ph.D. thesis research on the effects of rock type on alpine plant distribution and physiology. But much of the time, she hikes simply for leisure. Obsessively wanting to explore every bit of the Sierra, she has hiked thousands of on- and off-trail miles and climbed more than 600 peaks in the mountain range. Many of her wanderings are now directed to gather data for several Wilderness Press titles and to introduce her two young daughters to the wonders of the mountains. For them as well, Yosemite is rapidly becoming a favorite location.

Until recently a resident of Bishop, California, Wenk is currently living in Sydney, Australia, with her husband, Douglas, and daughters, Eleanor and Sophia. There she is working as a research fellow at Macquarie University and enjoying Australia's exquisite eucalyptus forests, vegetated slot canyons, and wonderful birdlife—except during the Northern Hemisphere summer, which she continues to spend exploring the Sierra.

OTHER TITLES BY ELIZABETH WENK

John Muir Trail (with Kathy Morey)

One Best Hike: Grand Canyon

One Best Hike: Mt. Whitney